Respiratory Disease Series: Diagnostic Tools and Disease Managements

Series Editors

Hiroyuki Nakamura, Professor Emeritus, Tokyo Medical University, Tokyo, Japan
Kazutetsu Aoshiba, Visiting Professor, Tokyo Medical University Ibaraki Medical Center, Ibaraki, Japan

This book series cover a variety of topics in respiratory diseases, with each volume providing an overview of the current state of knowledge, recent discoveries and future prospects for each disease. In each chapter the editors pose critical questions, which are often unresolved clinical issues. These are then discussed by the authors, providing insights and suggestions as to which developments need to be addressed. The series offers new information, which will inspire innovative ideas to further develop respiratory medicine. This collection of monographs is aimed at benefiting patients across the globe suffering from respiratory disease.

Edited by established authorities in the field and written by pioneering experts, this book series will be valuable to those researchers and physicians working in respiratory medicine. The series is aimed at a broad readership, and the books will also be a valuable resource for radiologists, emergency medicine physicians, pathologists, pharmacologists and basic research scientists.

Yasunari Miyazaki
Editor

Hypersensitivity Pneumonitis

Springer

Editor
Yasunari Miyazaki
Department of Respiratory Medicine
Tokyo Medical and Dental University
Bunkyo-ku, Tokyo, Japan

ISSN 2509-5552 ISSN 2509-5560 (electronic)
Respiratory Disease Series: Diagnostic Tools and Disease Managements
ISBN 978-981-96-7982-9 ISBN 978-981-96-7983-6 (eBook)
https://doi.org/10.1007/978-981-96-7983-6

This Springer imprint is published by the registered company Springer Nature Singapore Pte Ltd.
The registered company address is: 152 Beach Road, #21-01/04 Gateway East, Singapore 189721, Singapore

Contents

Part I
Definition, Epidemiology and Pathogenesis

Chapter 1
Disease Definition and Various Antigens

What Is the Definition and Causative Antigens of HP?

Yasunari Miyazaki

1 History of Hypersensitivity Pneumonitis

Hypersensitivity pneumonitis has a long history, including farmer's lung (1924), malt worker's lung (1928), and maple bark stripper's lung (1932). It was initially recognized as a pulmonary disease with acute respiratory symptoms as an occupational disease. First it was reported in the year 1932 by Campbell et al. as a disease caused by exposure to moldy hay in farmers [1]. Although it was not recognized as an allergic disease, in 1959, Pepys demonstrated the presence of precipitating antibodies to *Aspergillus* in the serum of patients suffering from malt workers' lungs and further demonstrated the presence of precipitating antibodies to thermophilic actinomycetes in the serum of patients suffering from farmer's lungs. As a result, hypersensitivity pneumonitis (acute, nonfibrotic) came to be recognized as an allergic disease to specific antigens [2]. On the other hand, the first report of chronic (fibrotic) hypersensitivity pneumonitis was published in 1968 by Seal et al. In a report of five cases of farmer's lung, three reported transitioning to chronic disease. Since then, there have been sporadic case reports of chronic hypersensitivity pneumonitis with farmer's lung disease and bird fancier's disease. Many cases of chronic hypersensitivity pneumonitis were reported in 1993 by Perez-Padilla R, Selman et al. [3] and Murayama, Yoshizawa et al. [4].

Y. Miyazaki (✉)
Department of Respiratory Medicine, Tokyo Medical and Dental University, Bunkyo-ku, Tokyo, Japan
e-mail: miyazaki.pilm@tmd.ac.jp

Y. Miyazaki (ed.), *Hypersensitivity Pneumonitis*, Respiratory Disease Series: Diagnostic Tools and Disease Managements,
https://doi.org/10.1007/978-981-96-7983-6_1

2 Disease Concept

Inciting antigens react with specific antibodies (type III allergy) or sensitized lymphocytes (type IV allergy) to form cellular bronchiolitis, lymphocytic alveolitis, and granuloma Th1 and Th17 reaction in sensitized individuals. However, in the chronic phase, this immune pathology changes as the immune response shifts from Th1 to Th2, depending on the type and amount of the causative antigen, the clearance rate in the lung, and internal and external factors. Fibrosis develops in the bronchiolar and centrilobular areas, resulting in interstitial lung disease with progressive fibrosis. The altered immune responses are implicated in fibrosis [5]. Analyses of the immune/allergic reactions of hypersensitivity pneumonitis, such as neutrophil reactions, lymphocyte reactions, and innate immunity of antigen-presenting cells after exposure to antigens, have progressed gradually. It is a future task to elucidate how it causes allergic inflammation and ultimately leads to fibrosis [6–8]. In recent years, analyses of MUC5b and telomeres have also revealed that there is a genetic predisposition to onset [9], and it has also been found that a single nucleotide polymorphism of TOLLIP is associated with disease progression [10]. The difficulty in diagnosing fibrotic hypersensitivity pneumonitis is thought to be due to the difficulty in finding antigens. Even now after the publication of international clinical guidelines [11, 12], we still rely on the "enthusiasm" of the attending physicians. Steady progress in immunology and genetics has led to "new light."

3 Causative Antigens

There are more than 300 inhaled antigens listed that can cause hypersensitivity pneumonitis, including bacteria, fungi, animal-derived proteins, and low-molecular-weight compounds. Representative antigens are shown in Table 1.1. It should be noted that the name of the subtype of the disease is based on the occupation and living conditions that indicate the environment of its onset and should not indicate the name of causative antigens. For example, farmer's lung is a disease that develops during dairy farming and working in pasture silos, and the causative antigens are bacteria, such as *Saccharopolyspora rectivirgula* and *Thermoactinomyces vulgaris*, but fungi, such as *Absidia*, *Eurotium*, and *Wallemia*, are thought to be causative in France. In other words, since bacteria and fungi inhabiting various countries, regions, and weather conditions are diverse, causative antigens also differ from country to country and region to region [13]. Summer-type hypersensitivity pneumonitis is a disease peculiar to Japan and is caused by a fungus (*Trichosporon*) that grows in old wooden houses against the backdrop of a hot and humid climate. Bird-related hypersensitivity pneumonitis includes bird fancier's lung caused by antigens contained in bird droppings and feathers, and also by feather products. Farmer's lung is caused by thermophilic actinomycetes growing in pasture grass, humidifier lung is caused by fungi and bacteria that grow in humidifier water tanks, and

Table 1.1 List of causative antigens of hypersensitivity pneumonitis

Subtype of hypersensitivity pneumonitis	Sources	Antigens
Bird-related hypersensitivity pneumonitis	Bird breeding	Bird droppings
	Birds' visit to home garden	Bird droppings
	Chicken manure fertilizer use	Bird droppings
	Stuffed bird	Feather
(Feather duvet lung)	Use of feather duvet	Feather
Farmer's lung	Dairy work	*Saccharopolyspora rectivirgula,*
		Themoactinomyces vulgaris, Absidia corymbifera,
		Eurotium amstelodami, Wallemia sebi
		Rhizopus spp.
Summer-type hypersensitivity pneumonitis	House	*Trichosporon asahii, T. dermatis*
Home-related hypersensitivity pneumonitis	House	*Candida albicans, Aspergillus niger, A.fumigatus*
		Cephalosporium acremonium, Fusarium napiforme
		Humicola fuscoatra, Peziza domiciliana
		Penicillium corylophilum,
Humidifier's lung	Use of humidifier	*Cladosporium* sp. *Aspergillus flavus? Phoma herbarum?*
Painter's lung	Car paint	Isocyanate
Mechanic's lung	Machine work	*Mycobacterium Immunogenum*
		Acinetobactor Iwoffii, Pseudomonas fluorescens
Flour lung	Confectionery	Flour
Coffee worker's lung	Coffee bean roasting	Coffee bean dust
Greenhouse grower's lung	Orchid cultivation in greenhouse	Fungi in wood chips
	Cucumber cultivation in greenhouse	Unknown
Mushroom grower's lung	Shiitake cultivation	Shiitake spores
	Enoki mushroom cultivation	Enoki mushroom spores
Cork lung	Cork manufacturing work	*Penicillium glabrum, A. fumigatus,*
		Chrysonilia sitophilia
Hot-tub lung	Hot tub, shower, mist	*Cladosporium,*
		Mycobacterium avium complex

mushroom grower's lung is caused by mushroom spores and fungi and bacteria that grow in the growing environment. The most important thing in diagnosing hypersensitivity pneumonitis is to identify the causative antigen. If the causative antigen can be identified, the cause can be eliminated and hence, cure can be expected. Therefore, in Japan, a reagent kit for measuring specific antibodies that can diagnose the causative antigen by serodiagnosis was developed. There are anti-*Trichosporon asahii* antibody measurement kits for diagnosing summer-type hypersensitivity pneumonitis, and bird-specific IgG antibody measurement kits for diagnosing bird-associated hypersensitivity pneumonitis.

References

1. Campbell J. Acute symptoms following work with hay. Br Med J. 1932;2:1143.
2. Pepys J, Riddell R, Citron K, Clayton Y. Precipitins against extracts of Hay and Moulds in the serum of patients with farmer's lung, Aspergillosis, asthma, and sarcoidosis. Thorax. 1962;17:366–74.
3. Perez-Padilla R, Salas J, Chapela R, Sanchez M, Carrillo G, Perez R, Sansores R, Gaxiola M, Selman M. Mortality in Mexican patients with chronic pigeon breeder's lung compared with those with usual interstitial pneumonia. Am Rev Respir Dis. 1993;148:49–53.
4. Murayama J, Yoshizawa Y, Ohtsuka M, Hasegawa S. Lung fibrosis in hypersensitivity pneumonitis. Association with CD4+ but not CD8+ cell dominant alveolitis and insidious onset. Chest. 1993;104:38–43.
5. Kishi M, Miyazaki Y, Jinta T, Furusawa H, Ohtani Y, Inase N, Yoshizawa Y. Pathogenesis of cBFL in common with IPF? Correlation of IP-10/TARC ratio with histological patterns. Thorax. 2008;63:810–6.
6. Mitaka K, Miyazaki Y, Yasui M, Furuie M, Miyake S, Inase N, Yoshizawa Y. Th2-biased immune responses are important in a murine model of chronic hypersensitivity pneumonitis. Int Arch Allergy Immunol. 2011;154:264–74.
7. Ishizuka M, Miyazaki Y, Masuo M, Suhara K, Tateishi T, Yasui M, Inase N. Interleukin-17A and neutrophils in a murine model of bird-related hypersensitivity pneumonitis. PLoS One. 2015;10:e0137978.
8. Daito H, Kikuchi T, Sakakibara T, Gomi K, Damayanti T, Zaini J, Tode N, Kanehira M, Koyama S, Fujimura S, Ebina M, Ishii KJ, Akira S, Takai T, Watanabe A, Nukiwa T. Mycobacterial hypersensitivity pneumonitis requires TLR9-MyD88 in lung CD11b+ CD11c+ cells. Eur Respir J. 2011;38:688–701.
9. Ley B, Newton CA, Arnould I, Elicker BM, Henry TS, Vittinghoff E, Golden JA, Jones KD, Batra K, Torrealba J, Garcia CK, Wolters PJ. The MUC5B promoter polymorphism and telomere length in patients with chronic hypersensitivity pneumonitis: an observational cohort-control study. Lancet Respir Med. 2017;5:639–47.
10. Katayanagi S, Setoguchi Y, Kitagawa S, Okamoto T, Miyazaki Y. Alternative gene expression by TOLLIP variant is associated with lung function in chronic hypersensitivity pneumonitis. Chest. 2022;161:458–69.
11. Raghu G, Remy-Jardin M, Ryerson CJ, Myers JL, Kreuter M, Vasakova M, Bargagli E, Chung JH, Collins BF, Bendstrup E, Chami HA, Chua AT, Corte TJ, Dalphin JC, Danoff SK, Diaz-Mendoza J, Duggal A, Egashira R, Ewing T, Gulati M, Inoue Y, Jenkins AR, Johannson KA, Johkoh T, Tamae-Kakazu M, Kitaichi M, Knight SL, Koschel D, Lederer DJ, Mageto Y, Maier LA, Matiz C, Morell F, Nicholson AG, Patolia S, Pereira CA, Renzoni EA, Salisbury ML, Selman M, SLF W, Wuyts WA, Wilson KC. Diagnosis of Hypersensitivity Pneumonitis in

Adults. An Official ATS/JRS/ALAT Clinical Practice Guideline. Am J Respir Crit Care Med. 2020;202:e36–69.

12. Fernandez Perez ER, Travis WD, Lynch DA, Brown KK, Johannson KA, Selman M, Ryu JH, Wells AU, Tony Huang YC, Pereira CAC, Scholand MB, Villar A, Inase N, Evans RB, Mette SA, Frazer-Green L. Diagnosis and evaluation of hypersensitivity pneumonitis: CHEST guideline and expert panel report. Chest. 2021;160:e97–e156.
13. Selman M, Lacasse Y, Pardo A, Cormier Y. Hypersensitivity pneumonitis caused by fungi. Proc Am Thorac Soc. 2010;7:229–36.

Chapter 2
Epidemiology, Clinical Features, and Clinical Subtypes in Acute/Chronic and Nonfibrotic/Fibrotic

What Is the Epidemiology of Hypersensitivity Pneumonitis in Japan and Other Countries?

Tsukasa Okamoto

1 Introduction

Hypersensitivity pneumonitis (HP) is an immunologically mediated lung disease resulting from inhalational exposure to a variety of antigens. The history of HP dates back to 1932, when Campbell et al. reported it as a disease caused by exposure to "moldy hay" in farm workers [1]. Initially, it was recognized as an occupational febrile disease, but epidemiologic studies began in the late 1950s, and it was revealed to be an allergic disease. In Japan, sugarcane lung, farmer's lung, bird-fancier's lung, and mushroom worker's lung were reported since the late 1960s. Furthermore, *Trichosporon* species was found to be the cause of summer-type HP, which is common in Japan [2–4].

There are more than 300 known causative antigens, and the number is increasing each year [5]. Inhalant antigens associated with occupational exposure and those present in the daily living environment, such as bird-related HP and home-related HP, are also recognized. Potential sources of inciting antigen vary among geographic regions and are influenced by multiple climatic, cultural, socioeconomic, and occupational factors [6].

Until a couple of years ago, HP was divided into two forms, namely, acute and chronic HP, and it was initially thought that only a relatively small number of cases were fibrotic. However, it became increasingly clear that the clinical picture of fibrotic HP was similar to that of idiopathic pulmonary fibrosis (IPF), and it attracted attention as a differential disease for IPF.

T. Okamoto (✉)
Division of Integrated Facilities, Center for Personalized Medicine for Healthy Aging, Institute of Science Tokyo, Tokyo, Japan
e-mail: tokamoto.pulm@tmd.ac.hp

Y. Miyazaki (ed.), *Hypersensitivity Pneumonitis*, Respiratory Disease Series: Diagnostic Tools and Disease Managements,
https://doi.org/10.1007/978-981-96-7983-6_2

Although HP is one of the most common types of interstitial lung diseases (ILDs), a limited number of studies have focused on its epidemiology. Due to the increasing number of HP diagnoses, previous reports on epidemiological studies are summarized in this chapter.

2 Clinical Subtypes

Historically, HP was classified into acute and chronic according to the clinical presentations, and chronic HP was further subgrouped into recurrent type and insidious type (Fig. 2.1). Patients with recurrent chronic HP have recurrent but gradually diminished acute episodes, including mild dyspnea on exertion, cough, and low-grade fever. However, patients with insidious chronic HP have a slowly progressive course without acute episodes [7]. The diagnosis of patients with acute HP is relatively simple when they have acute episodes and have typical high-resolution computed tomography (HRCT) findings. Although some develop an acute HP with resolution of disease with removal from exposure, a subgroup of subjects may experience chronic HP, leading to increased mortality. A subset of subjects with chronic HP develops fibrotic HP, characterized clinically by the presence of pulmonary fibrosis [5, 8]. On the other hand, distinguishing chronic HP from IPF and other fibrosing ILDs is extremely difficult because of similar clinical, radiological, and pathological features among these diseases [9].

However, these categories are not easy to demarcate and in many studies, the demarcation has been variable and arbitrary. Since the presence or absence of radiographic or histopathological fibrosis is the major determinant of prognosis [10–13], the guideline from ATS/JRS/ALAT and CHEST categorized HP as either fibrotic (i.e., mixed inflammatory plus fibrotic or purely fibrotic) or nonfibrotic (i.e., purely inflammatory), given the greater clinical utility of this stratification [5, 8].

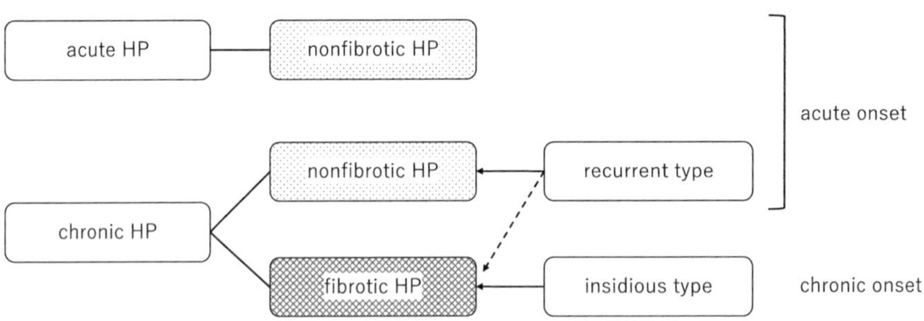

Fig. 2.1 Classification of hypersensitivity pneumonitis

3 Epidemiology

The proportion of HP among all ILD cases varies tremendously, ranging from 2% to 47% in studies and registries [14–19]. According to these data, the relative frequency of HP was higher in Asia, particularly in India (10.7–47.3%) and Pakistan (12.3%), compared to most of the North American (only 2%) and European cohorts [16, 17, 20–22]. Furthermore, evidence has shown that the HP diagnosis has increased in recent years. An important study highlights the importance of occult exposure as a cause of disease and the ability of HP to mimic IPF [23]. In that study, 60 consecutive patients diagnosed with diagnosis of IPF were prospectively followed up for 6 years. Almost half of the patients were subsequently diagnosed with chronic HP, and most of these cases were attributed to exposure to occult avian antigens from commonly used feather bedding. Additionally, epidemiologic studies recently reported from the United States show a cumulative incidence rate of 1.3–1.9 per 100,000 persons and an annual prevalence rate of 1.6–2.7 per 100,000 persons, with an upward trend [24]. However, the disease definitions, study designs, and ascertainment of incident versus prevalent cases were different [4, 24–33]. As a precaution, in many reports, fibrosis and nonfibrosis are not reported separately. Therefore, further investigations are needed to clarify the incidence and prevalence of HP. Now I will present epidemiological studies by regions, including Japan at first (Table 2.1) followed by other countries (Tables 2.2 and 2.3).

3.1 Japan

There are several epidemiological studies in Japan. The frequencies of HP by cause according to the national survey of HP are shown in Table 2.1. The first national survey of HP in Japan was reported in 1991 [2]. A total of 835 cases of acute HP was recognized from 1980 to 1989. Summer-type HP, which is induced by inhalation of seasonal mold, *Trichosporon asahii*, was reported to be the most prevalent (81.9% of 331 cases) and bird fancier's lung accounted for only 5.7% of cases.

A subsequent national survey conducted in 1999 focused on chronic HP, and the report covered 36 cases of chronic HP, including summer-type HP (n = 10, 28%), bird fancier's lung (n = 7, 20%), home-related HP (n = 5, 14%), isocyanate-induced HP (n = 5, 14%), farmer's lung (n = 4, 11%), and other variants of the disease (n = 5, 14%) [27].

In the second national survey of chronic HP, we collected 222 cases diagnosed during the 10-year period from 2000 to 2009 from all over Japan. These included 134 cases of bird-related HP, 33 cases of summer-type HP, 25 cases of home-related HP, 4 cases of farmer's lung, 3 cases of isocyanate-induced HP, and 23 other cases. While occupational HP such as farmer's lung and isocyanate-induced HP decreased, the proportion of

Table 2.1 Japanese nationwide studies

Type	Number	%
Reported in 1991		
Summer-type HP	621	74.4
Farmer's lung	68	8.1
Humidifier lung	36	4.3
Bird fancier's lung	34	4.1
Others	19	2.3
Unknown	57	6.8
Total	835	100
Reported in 1999		
Summer-type HP	10	27.8
Bird fancier's lung	7	19.4
Isocyanate-induced HP	5	13.9
Home-related HP	5	13.9
Farmer's lung	4	11.1
Others	5	13.9
Total	36	100
Reported in 2013		
Bird-related HP	134	60.4
Summer-type HP	33	14.9
Home-related HP	25	11.3
Farmer's lung	4	1.8
Isocyanate-induced HP	3	1.4
Others	23	10.4
Total	222	100

The numbers and proportions are shown. *HP* hypersensitivity pneumonitis

Table 2.2 Incidence and prevalence of hypersensitivity pneumonitis

Country		Time	
North America			
United States	Incidence	2004–2013	1.28–1.94
United States	Prevalence	2004–2013	1.67–2.71
Europe			
Belgium	Incidence	1992–1996	0.12
Belgium	Prevalence	1992–1996	0.81
Greece	Incidence	2004	0.13
Greece	Prevalence	2004	0.45
France	Incidence	2012	0.9
France	Prevalence	2012	2.3
Six countries[a]	Incidence	2018	0.3–3.2
Six countries[a]	Prevalence	2018	6.2–12.3

Incidence and prevalence defined as cases per 100,000

[a]Six countries consisted of Belgium, Denmark, Finland, Greece, Norway, and Portugal

Table 2.3 Relative frequencies of hypersensitivity pneumonitis in interstitial lung diseases

Country	Total number		Time	HP number (%)
North America				
United States	202	Incident cases	1988–1990	3 (1.5)
Canada	52	n/a	2006–2013	1 (1.9)
Canada	1285	n/a	2016–2017	97 (7.5)
Europe				
Belgium	264	Incident cases	1992–1996	32 (12.1)
Belgium	362	Prevalent cases	1992–1996	47 (13.0)
Belgium	464	Incident cases	2017–2019	58 (12.5%)
Greece	259	Incident cases	2004	7 (2.7)
Greece	967	Prevalent cases	2004	25 (2.6)
Denmark	431	Incident cases	2003–2009	32 (7.4)
Spain	511	Incident cases	2000–2001	34 (6.6)
Italy	3152	n/a	1998–2005	93 (2.9)
France	848	Prevalent cases	2012	28 (3.3)
Asia				
Turkey	2245	Incident cases	2007–2009	82 (3.7)
India	566	Incident cases	2015–2017	69 (12.2)
India	803	Prevalent cases	2015–2017	86 (10.7)
India	1084	Incident cases	2012–2015	513 (47.3)
Pakistan	253	n/a	2016–2018	31 (12.3)
China	1945	Incident cases	2012–2017	59 (3.0)
China	2615	Prevalent cases	2000–2012	62 (2.4)
Other				
Saudi Arabia	330	Incident case	2009–2011	21 (6.3)
Australia	705	n/a	2016–2019	66 (9.4)

n/a not applicable

bird-related HP increased, accounting for 60% of the cases. The reason why bird-related antigens are the most common causative antigens of fibrotic HP is thought to be due to the increasing recognition of the disease itself, the patient's own bird-feeding, as well as prolonged unawareness of antigen exposure, including the use of down products, neighbors' bird-keeping, wild birds in the surrounding environment, and poultry manure, and antigen specificity (reduced turnover of antigen in the lung area). Another factor is thought to be the general lack of testing tools, with the exception of summer-type HP and bird-related HP. The number of reports of farmer's lung and isocyanate-induced HP may have decreased due to improvements in the work environment. Regarding regional characteristics, bird-related HP was similar throughout Japan, while summer-type HP and home-related HP were seen in a few cases in northern Japan. The median proportion of lymphocytes in bronchoalveolar lavage fluid was high (24.5%). The primary findings of high-resolution computed tomography (HRCT) were ground-glass attenuation and interlobular septal thickening. Centrilobular fibrosis was the major pathological finding on examination of surgical lung biopsy specimens from 93 patients. The median survival time was 83 months.

Recently, we described the epidemiology of HP using the Japanese Diagnostic Procedure Combination database that includes data from 1031 hospitals [6]. In total, 3634 patients with HP were identified, including summer-type HP ($n = 490$), bird fancier's lung ($n = 199$), ventilation pneumonitis ($n = 106$), farmer's lung ($n = 48$), and unspecified HP ($n = 2761$). In-hospital mortality was significantly associated with old age ($p < 0.001$), low body mass index ($p = 0.016$), severe dyspnea ($p < 0.001$), and interestingly, bird-fancier's lung diagnosis on admission ($p = 0.031$).

3.2 United States

Recently, Fernández Pérez et al. have presented the annual incidence and prevalence using U.S. administrative claims-based data [24]. Between 2004 and 2013, the 1-year cumulative incidence rates ranged from 1.28 to 1.94 per 100,000 persons, and the 1-year prevalence rates for HP ranged from 1.67 to 2.71 per 100,000 persons. HP was more common among women and those older than 65 years. Most cases were classified as chronic HP. Approximately one-fourth met a criterion for fibrotic HP, which was associated with a higher mortality rate.

Another study was performed in southeast of United States and identified 261 patients with chronic HP; this was confirmed in clinic notes by a pulmonologist or an allergist [34]. Interestingly, an estimated prevalence rate in this area was higher 6.5 per 100,000 persons compared to the previous report in Unites States. An exposure source was mentioned in 69.3% of the patient and the most common sources were environmental molds (43.1%) and birds (26.0%).

3.3 Europe

One of first prospective registry studies evaluated the epidemiology in Flanders, the north region of Belgium between 1992 and 1996 [25]. A total of 362 cases were recruited from 20 centers. The frequency of HP was 13% and the majority (75%) were associated with pigeon breeding.

In Greece, a similar distribution of ILD subtypes was observed [16]. In a multicenter ILD registry study, 967 patients were recruited from pulmonary divisions across the country. The prevalence of HP was relatively low (2.6%).

A Danish study that sought to describe the incidence of ILDs in central Denmark recruited 431 patients from a single center between 2003 and 2009 [20]. Cases were adjudicated by multidisciplinary discussion (MDD). The most common ILD was IPF (28%), followed by CTD-ILD (12.5%) and HP (7%).

In Spain, a multicenter registry study that enrolled patients via surveys completed by 23 pulmonary medicine clinics between 2000 and 2001 noted the most common ILD was IPF (38.6%) and HP was 6.6% [18]. Similar to observations from the Belgium cohort, pigeon breeding was the most common exposure.

In Italy, 3152 patients were enrolled via surveys completed by 79 centers across 20 regions [35]. Sarcoidosis was the most frequently reported ILD (33.7%), followed by IPF (27.4%). The frequency of HP was as low as 2.9%.

In France, a study that described the population burden of chronic ILDs among people living in Seine-Saint-Denis, a multi-ethnic urbanized area of Greater Paris, reviewed a total 848 cases and validated centrally by MDD [36]. There was a low prevalence of HP (3.3%).

Epidemiological study of ILDs in six European countries, including Belgium, Denmark, Finland, Greece, Norway, and Portugal, presents national data for 2018. The incidence of HP ranged from 0.3 to 3.2 per 100,000 people, with a prevalence of 1.9 to 14.3 per 100,000 people [37].

Nasser et al. conducted a longitudinal, retrospective cohort study using administrative claims data from the French national administrative healthcare database, which identified a total of 14,413 patients with progressive fibrosing ILD (PF-ILD) [38]. The main diagnostic categories represented were exposure-related ILD other than HP (24.2%) including coal workers' pneumoconiosis, asbestosis, pneumoconiosis due to other dust containing silica, and so on. The percentage of HP was only 5.1%.

Although there was only limited number of reports, which showed the frequency of fibrotic and nonfibrotic HP in accordance with recent guidelines, recent epidemiologic study in Belgium identified 58 (12.5%) of HP cases and features of fibrosis were identified in 81% of patients with HP [39].

3.4 Asia

Compared to Europe and North America, the English language literature on ILD in Asia has until recently been quite limited. In the last decade, several epidemiologic studies evaluating relative frequency of ILDs have emerged from Turkey, India, Pakistan, and China.

In India, a few large database studies have evaluated the epidemiology of ILD in 2018. The frequency of HP was 10.7%. Of the patients with HP, the most common exposure was farming (59.3%), followed by bird feathers (15.1%). The second epidemiologic study in India involved a multicenter cohort study, which recruited 1084 patients with ILDs from 27 centers between 2012 and 2015 [17]. HP was the final diagnosis in majority of cases (47.3%). Among patients with HP, 48.1% had been exposed to air coolers, 26.3% to air conditioners, 21.4% to birds, and 20.7% to mold in their homes. Unlike other countries, air coolers and air conditioners were found to be the most common causative antigen in India. Of a total of 2005 ILD patients enrolled from 2015 to 2020, HP accounted for 14.4% [22]. HP is much more frequent in India (incidence, 1.4–2.9; prevalence, 6.2–12.3 per 100,000 population) compared to developed countries. In Pakistan, next to India, HP accounted 17.7% of a total of 744 patients with ILDs [40].

In China, two studies examined the epidemiology of ILD. The first study identified 1945 patients between 2012 and 2017 retrospectively [41]. The most common ILD subtype was IPF (20.3%), followed by CTD-ILD (18.3%). Only 3% of patients were diagnosed with HP. The most common exposure was mold followed by farming and birds. The second study evaluated the distribution of ILD among 2615 patients between 2000 and 2012 retrospectively [42]. Also, IPF was the most common subtype (26.5%), followed by CTD-ILD (24.1%). Only 2.4% of patients were identified as HP.

In the middle east, one study examined the frequency of ILD subtypes in Saudi Arabia prospectively from a single center between 2008 and 2011 [19]. A total of 330 patients were enrolled in this study and HP was identified in 6.3% of total. The most common exposure was birds identified in 66.7% of cases.

In Australia, a total of 1061 patients were recruited from four ILD centers across the continent between 2016 and 2019 [43]. The most common diagnosis was IPF (34%), followed by CTD-ILD (17.7%) and HP (9.4%).

4 Epidemiological Data by Causative Antigen

The antigens responsible for the disease in other countries vary widely depending on the mechanism, lifestyle, housing, and work environment. For example, farmer's lung caused by thermophilic actinomycetes species and summer-type HP caused by *Trichosporon* species tend to occur in hot and humid environments. The prevalence of farmer's lung is reported to be 420–3000 per 100,000 persons in the United States, 12–2300 in the United Kingdom, 4370 in France, and 1400–1700 in Finland, but is rare in Brazil and varies from country to country [44]. Summer-type HP is rare in Europe and the United States, and most cases have been reported from Japan. In occupational HP, the causative antigen varies depending on the industry in each country.

While bird-related HP was seen nationwide in Japan, it is also common overseas. In a report from the Mayo Clinic in the United States, the causative antigen was identified in 64 (75%) of 85 cases of HP (including acute and chronic cases): avian antigen in 34%, *Mycobacterium avium* complex in hot tub lung in 21%, abundant lung in 11%, and molds in dwellings in 9%. *Mycobacterium avium* complex in hot tub lung was found in 34% of cases [45]. A scoping review was performed to identify all publications describing HP cases and their associated exposures from 1990 to 2020 [46]. In assessed 967 publications, birds were the most common causative antigen (32%), followed by molds (17%).

5 Occupational HP and HP in Antigen-Exposed Individuals

Identification of the offending agent/source of exposure and removal from exposure to the causal workplace agent is also crucial in occupational HP. Barber et al. estimated the reported incidence of occupational HP in the UK between 1996 and 2015 using national reporting data [47]. There were 202 cases of occupational HP reported and the annual UK incidence was calculated as 1.4 per million workers. The mean age of cases was 52 years and cases were four times more likely to be men than women.

During the period studied, the common causes of occupational HP in the UK were exposures to metalworking fluids (35%), farming (17%), and birds (11%).

The few published cohort studies of occupational HP reported incidence rates of 2–5 cases per 10,000 farmers per year during the 1980s [48, 49]. Cross-sectional studies provided prevalence estimates in various high-risk workforces, such as workers exposed to tobacco (5.2%) [50], mollusk shells (23%) [51], isocyanates (0.9–4.7%) [52, 53], contaminated air conditioner (15%) [54], swimming pools (27%) [55], and metalworking fluids (5.6%) [56]. In farmers, farmer's lung developed in about 9% of farmers in humid areas of France and about 2% in dry areas of Scotland [31, 57]. The estimated prevalence rates of occupational HP ranged from 1.3% to 12.9% among farmers [26, 57–60] and from 8.0% to 10.4% among pigeon breeders [61, 62]. These data, however, usually come from reports of outbreak investigations, and it should be kept in mind that this often occurs in time- and place-limited epidemics.

For bird-related HP, HP was reported to occur in 6–20% of pigeon breeders and 0.5–7.5% of parrot breeders [30, 62, 63]. The hazard ratio for pigeon keepers was 14.36. In contrast, several reports pointed to a lower HP prevalence in smokers due to the immune impairment induced by smoking [28, 44, 64, 65].

6 Seasonal Variability

Seasonal variations of HP (especially, recurrent type) are recognized. Summer-type HP is more common during the hot and humid summer season, especially in western Japan. Acute summer-type HP peaks in July and 80% of all cases occur between June and September, and is rare in winter. As for bird-related HP, some cases develop or worsen in winter due to the use of down products such as down quilts and down jackets, and the increase in the number of migratory birds. Thus, some cases may have recurring respiratory symptoms seasonally each year, which should be carefully monitored during the clinical interview. Measurement of serum Krebs von den Lungen-6 (KL-6) and surfactant protein D (SP-D) is widely accepted in Japan, as a diagnostic test for interstitial lung diseases (ILDs) and as a marker of disease activity [66, 67]. In our experience of patients with summer-type HP, serum KL-6 and SP-D levels increase together with disease activity in hot and humid times of year, when *Trichosporon asahii* and other causative molds grow best. Conversely, patients with bird-related HP seem to present with higher serum levels of KL-6 and SP-D in winter [68, 69].

7 Genetic Factors

Familial aggregation of HP has been known for a long time, with the first report of two families with bird breeder's lung in 1975 [70]. In a study of fibrotic HP, 17.5% of patients with fibrotic HP had a familial history of ILDs in the first degree of consanguinity, confirming a familial clustering [71]. The familial history of this disease was suspected to be hereditary, since the cases were not from the same environment. Patients with a familial history of ILDs had a significantly younger age of onset compared to patients with an isolated case (57.5 vs. 64 years). Similarly, in a report in which family history was collected by questionnaire, 174 of the 1164 cases (15%) of all ILDs had a family history of ILDs and 10 cases (12%) of 87 HP cases had a family history of ILDs [72].

Several genes have been investigated as predictors of progression in fibrotic ILDs. In IPF, genome-wide association studies (GWASs) have identified several polymorphisms that are associated with the condition, including genes involved in telomere maintenance, mucin production, and the innate immune response. Ley et al. measured two single-nucleotide polymorphisms known to be associated with IPF (in MUC5B and TOLLIP) in two cohorts of patients with chronic HP ($n = 145$ and $n = 72$) [73]. In chronic HP, rs35705950 single-nucleotide polymorphism (SNP) in MUC5B promoter was associated with moderate-to-severe fibrosis and traction bronchiectasis on CT. Unlike in patients with IPF where this SNP is associated with improved survival, in chronic HP, the presence of the minor allele had no significant association with survival, although trended toward worse mortality (adjusted HR 2.01, $p = 0.063$). Similarly, we demonstrated that the rs5743899 SNP in TOLLIP was associated with rapid deterioration in FVC over time [74]. The potential role of telomere dysfunction in chronic HP was further investigated, which investigated the frequency and effect of mutations in telomere maintenance genes on survival in chronic HP [75].

8 Pediatric Cases

The first pediatric case was described in 1967 [76]. HP is a rare disease in childhood with the prevalence of 4 cases per million children and an incidence of 2 cases per year [77]. The average age of diagnosis at pediatric age is approximately 10 years. Ninety-five percent of the cases were males [78]. Mostly, the causative antigen is bird antigens in children. Specifically, childhood HP is often associated with exposure to antigens in the home environment or related to specific hobbies [79]. Children's ILDs, sometimes calls chILD, are increasingly recognized. Childhood HP is uncommon but may represent 50% of all chILDs [80–83]. Twenty-three children with confirmed pediatric HP were identified in German cohort [82]. Seven of the 23 children already had a chronic disease state at presentation. Of note, chILD occurs more frequently at a younger age and in boys.

In another study, the Australasian Registry Network for Orphan Lung Disease (ARNOLD) has identified problems in estimating rare disease prevalence; focusing on chILD in immunocompetent patients, a period prevalence of 1.5 cases per million children and a mortality rate of 7% were determined [84]. However, HP was not detected in this cohort.

Genetic factors including HLA-DR7, HLA-B8, and HLA-DQw3 may play an important role as 25% of children have a positive family history [85].

9 Conclusions

I have summarized the epidemiologic data of HP around the world and demonstrated that there is significant geographic heterogeneity. These differences may represent true differences based on demographics and exposures of the source populations or methodological differences in patient recruitment and disease classification. The number of cases of HP is expected to increase, since the diagnosis of HP was standardized by the guidelines. Epidemiological information based on globally standardized disease classification and diagnosis is needed.

References

1. Campbell J. Acute symptoms following work with hay. Br Med J. 1932;11:1143–4.
2. Ando M, Arima K, Yoneda R, Tamura M. Japanese summer-type hypersensitivity pneumonitis. Geographic distribution, home environment, and clinical characteristics of 621 cases. Am Rev Respir Dis. 1991;144:765–9.
3. Ando M, Suga M, Nishiura Y, Miyajima M. Summer-type hypersensitivity pneumonitis. Intern Med. 1995;34:707–12.
4. Okamoto T, Miyazaki Y, Ogura T, Chida K, Kohno N, Kohno S, Taniguchi H, Akagawa S, Mochizuki Y, Yamauchi K, Takahashi H, Johkoh T, Homma S, Kishi K, Ikushima S, Konno S, Mishima M, Ohta K, Nishioka Y, Yoshimura N, Munakata M, Watanabe K, Miyashita Y, Inase N. Nationwide epidemiological survey of chronic hypersensitivity pneumonitis in Japan. Respir Investig. 2013;51:191–9.
5. Raghu G, Remy-Jardin M, Ryerson CJ, Myers JL, Kreuter M, Vasakova M, Bargagli E, Chung JH, Collins BF, Bendstrup E, Chami HA, Chua AT, Corte TJ, Dalphin JC, Danoff SK, Diaz-Mendoza J, Duggal A, Egashira R, Ewing T, Gulati M, Inoue Y, Jenkins AR, Johannson KA, Johkoh T, Tamae-Kakazu M, Kitaichi M, Knight SL, Koschel D, Lederer DJ, Mageto Y, Maier LA, Matiz C, Morell F, Nicholson AG, Patolia S, Pereira CA, Renzoni EA, Salisbury ML, Selman M, SLF W, Wuyts WA, Wilson KC. Diagnosis of hypersensitivity pneumonitis in adults. An official ATS/JRS/ALAT clinical practice guideline. Am J Respir Crit Care Med. 2020;202:e36–69.
6. Yamashita S, Okamoto T, Kawahara T, Tateishi T, Anzai T, Takahashi K, Fushimi K, Miyazaki Y. Database analysis of hypersensitivity pneumonitis in Japan. Respir Investig. 2023;61:172–80.
7. Ohtani Y, Saiki S, Sumi Y, Inase N, Miyake S, Costabel U, Yoshizawa Y. Clinical features of recurrent and insidious chronic bird fancier's lung. Ann Allergy Asthma Immunol. 2003;90:604–10.
8. Fernández Pérez ER, Travis WD, Lynch DA, Brown KK, Johannson KA, Selman M, Ryu JH, Wells AU, Tony Huang YC, Pereira CAC, Scholand MB, Villar A, Inase N, Evans RB, Mette SA, Frazer-Green L. Diagnosis and evaluation of hypersensitivity pneumonitis: CHEST guideline and expert panel report. Chest. 2021;160:e97–e156.
9. Pérez-Padilla R, Salas J, Chapela R, Sánchez M, Carrillo G, Pérez R, Sansores R, Gaxiola M, Selman M. Mortality in Mexican patients with chronic pigeon breeder's lung compared with those with usual interstitial pneumonia. Am Rev Respir Dis. 1993;148:49–53.
10. Churg A, Sin DD, Everett D, Brown K, Cool C. Pathologic patterns and survival in chronic hypersensitivity pneumonitis. Am J Surg Pathol. 2009;33:1765–70.
11. Mooney JJ, Elicker BM, Urbania TH, Agarwal MR, Ryerson CJ, Nguyen MLT, Woodruff PG, Jones KD, Collard HR, King TE Jr, Koth LL. Radiographic fibrosis score predicts survival in hypersensitivity pneumonitis. Chest. 2013;144:586–92.

12. Salisbury ML, Gu T, Murray S, Gross BH, Chughtai A, Sayyouh M, Kazerooni EA, Myers JL, Lagstein A, Konopka KE, Belloli EA, Sheth JS, White ES, Holtze C, Martinez FJ, Flaherty KR. Hypersensitivity pneumonitis: radiologic phenotypes are associated with distinct survival time and pulmonary function trajectory. Chest. 2019;155:699–711.
13. Chiba S, Tsuchiya K, Akashi T, Ishizuka M, Okamoto T, Furusawa H, Tateishi T, Kishino M, Miyazaki Y, Tateishi U, Takemura T, Inase N. Chronic hypersensitivity pneumonitis with a usual interstitial pneumonia-like pattern: correlation between histopathologic and clinical findings. Chest. 2016;149:1473–81.
14. Thomeer MJ, Costabe U, Rizzato G, Poletti V, Demedts M. Comparison of registries of interstitial lung diseases in three European countries. Eur Respir J Suppl. 2001;32:114s–8s.
15. Kreuter M, Herth FJ, Wacker M, Leidl R, Hellmann A, Pfeifer M, Behr J, Witt S, Kauschka D, Mall M, Günther A, Markart P. Exploring clinical and epidemiological characteristics of interstitial lung diseases: rationale, aims, and design of a nationwide prospective registry–The EXCITING-ILD registry. Biomed Res Int. 2015;2015:123876.
16. Karakatsani A, Papakosta D, Rapti A, Antoniou KM, Dimadi M, Markopoulou A, Latsi P, Polychronopoulos V, Birba G, Ch L, Bouros D. Epidemiology of interstitial lung diseases in Greece. Respir Med. 2009;103:1122–9.
17. Singh S, Collins BF, Sharma BB, Joshi JM, Talwar D, Katiyar S, Singh N, Ho L, Samaria JK, Bhattacharya P, Gupta R, Chaudhari S, Singh T, Moond V, Pipavath S, Ahuja J, Chetambath R, Ghoshal AG, Jain NK, Devi HJ, Kant S, Koul P, Dhar R, Swarnakar R, Sharma SK, Roy DJ, Sarmah KR, Jankharia B, Schmidt R, Katiyar SK, Jindal A, Mangal DK, Singh V, Raghu G. Interstitial lung disease in India. Results of a prospective registry. Am J Respir Crit Care Med. 2017;195:801–13.
18. Xaubet A, Ancochea J, Morell F, Rodriguez-Arias JM, Villena V, Blanquer R, Montero C, Sueiro A, Disdier C, Vendrell M. Report on the incidence of interstitial lung diseases in Spain. Sarcoidosis Vasc Diffuse Lung Dis. 2004;21:64–70.
19. Alhamad EH. Interstitial lung diseases in Saudi Arabia: a single-center study. Ann Thorac Med. 2013;8:33–7.
20. Hyldgaard C, Hilberg O, Muller A, Bendstrup E. A cohort study of interstitial lung diseases in Central Denmark. Respir Med. 2014;108:793–9.
21. Singh S, Collins BF, Bairwa M, Joshi JM, Talwar D, Singh N, Samaria JK, Mangal DK, Singh V, Raghu G. Hypersensitivity pneumonitis and its correlation with ambient air pollution in urban India. Eur Respir J. 2019;53:1801563.
22. Dhooria S, Sehgal IS, Agarwal R, Muthu V, Prasad KT, Kathirvel S, Garg M, Bal A, Aggarwal AN, Behera D. Incidence, prevalence, and national burden of interstitial lung diseases in India: estimates from two studies of 3089 subjects. PLoS One. 2022;17:e0271665.
23. Morell F, Villar A, Montero M, Muñoz X, Colby TV, Pipvath S, Cruz MJ, Raghu G. Chronic hypersensitivity pneumonitis in patients diagnosed with idiopathic pulmonary fibrosis: a prospective case-cohort study. Lancet Respir Med. 2013;1:685–94.
24. Fernández Pérez ER, Kong AM, Raimundo K, Koelsch TL, Kulkarni R, Cole AL. Epidemiology of hypersensitivity pneumonitis among an insured population in the United States: a claims-based cohort analysis. Ann Am Thorac Soc. 2018;15:460–9.
25. Thomeer M, Demedts M, Vandeurzen K. Registration of interstitial lung diseases by 20 centres of respiratory medicine in Flanders. Acta Clin Belg. 2001;56:163–72.
26. Depierre A, Dalphin JC, Pernet D, Dubiez A, Faucompré C, Breton JL. Epidemiological study of farmer's lung in five districts of the French Doubs province. Thorax. 1988;43:429–35.
27. Yoshizawa Y, Ohtani Y, Hayakawa H, Sato A, Suga M, Ando M. Chronic hypersensitivity pneumonitis in Japan: a nationwide epidemiologic survey. J Allergy Clin Immunol. 1999;103:315–20.
28. Solaymani-Dodaran M, West J, Smith C, Hubbard R. Extrinsic allergic alveolitis: incidence and mortality in the general population. QJM. 2007;100:233–7.
29. Kornum JB, Christensen S, Grijota M, Pedersen L, Wogelius P, Beiderbeck A, Sørensen HT. The incidence of interstitial lung disease 1995-2005: a Danish nationwide population-based study. BMC Pulm Med. 2008;8:24.

30. Hendrick DJ, Faux JA, Marshall R. Budgerigar-fancier's lung: the commonest variety of allergic alveolitis in Britain. Br Med J. 1978;2:81–4.
31. Grant IW, Blyth W, Wardrop VE, Gordon RM, Pearson JC, Mair A. Prevalence of farmer's lung in Scotland: a pilot survey. Br Med J. 1972;1:530–4.
32. Christensen LT, Schmidt CD, Robbins L. Pigeon breeders' disease–a prevalence study and review. Clin Allergy. 1975;5:417–30.
33. Fenclová Z, Pelclová D, Urban P, Navrátil T, Klusácková P, Lebedová J. Occupational hypersensitivity pneumonitis reported to the Czech National Registry of Occupational Diseases in the period 1992-2005. Ind Health. 2009;47:443–8.
34. Gu JP, Tsai CL, Wysham NG, Huang YT. Chronic hypersensitivity pneumonitis in the southeastern United States: an assessment of how clinicians reached the diagnosis. BMC Pulm Med. 2020;20:32.
35. Tinelli C, De Silvestri A, Richeldi L, Oggionni T. The Italian register for diffuse infiltrative lung disorders (RIPID): a four-year report. Sarcoidosis Vasc Diffuse Lung Dis. 2005;22 Suppl 1:S4–8.
36. Duchemann B, Annesi-Maesano I, Jacobe de Naurois C, Sanyal S, Brillet PY, Brauner M, Kambouchner M, Huynh S, Naccache JM, Borie R, Piquet J, Mekinian A, Virally J, Uzunhan Y, Cadranel J, Crestani B, Fain O, Lhote F, Dhote R, Saidenberg-Kermanac'h N, Rosental PA, Valeyre D, Nunes H. Prevalence and incidence of interstitial lung diseases in a multi-ethnic county of Greater Paris. Eur Respir J. 2017;50:1602419.
37. Hilberg O, Hoffmann-Vold AM, Smith V, Bouros D, Kilpeläinen M, Guiot J, Morais A, Clemente S, Daniil Z, Papakosta D, Fretheim H, Neves S, Alfaro TM, Antoniou KM, Valveny N, Asijee G, Soulard S, Wuyts W. Epidemiology of interstitial lung diseases and their progressive-fibrosing behaviour in six European countries. ERJ Open Res. 2022;8:8.
38. Nasser M, Larrieu S, Boussel L, Si-Mohamed S, Bazin F, Marque S, Massol J, Thivolet-Bejui F, Chalabreysse L, Maucort-Boulch D, Hachulla E, Jouneau S, Le Lay K, Cottin V. Estimates of epidemiology, mortality and disease burden associated with progressive fibrosing interstitial lung disease in France (the PROGRESS study). Respir Res. 2021;22:162.
39. Gagliardi M, Berg DV, Heylen CE, Koenig S, Hoton D, Tamirou F, Pieters T, Ghaye B, Froidure A. Real-life prevalence of progressive fibrosing interstitial lung diseases. Sci Rep. 2021;11:23988.
40. Zubairi ABS, Ansarie M, Mahmud T, Ashraf S, Rao NA, Javaid A, Shaheen Z, Khan S, Khan A. National registry of interstitial lung disease from Pakistan. Cureus. 2021;13:e14684.
41. Guo B, Wang L, Xia S, Mao M, Qian W, Peng X, Zheng Z, Chen R, Han Q, Luo Q. The interstitial lung disease spectrum under a uniform diagnostic algorithm: a retrospective study of 1,945 individuals. J Thorac Dis. 2020;12:3688–96.
42. Ban C, Yan W, Xie B, Zhu M, Liu Y, Zhang S, Ye Q, Ren Y, Jiang D, Geng J, Dai H, Wang C. Spectrum of interstitial lung disease in China from 2000 to 2012. Eur Respir J. 2018;52:1701554.
43. Moore I, Wrobel J, Rhodes J, Lin Q, Webster S, Jo H, Troy L, Grainge C, Glaspole I, Corte TJ. Australasian interstitial lung disease registry (AILDR): objectives, design and rationale of a bi-national prospective database. BMC Pulm Med. 2020;20:257.
44. Pereira CA, Gimenez A, Kuranishi L, Storrer K. Chronic hypersensitivity pneumonitis. J Asthma Allergy. 2016;9:171–81.
45. Hanak V, Golbin JM, Ryu JH. Causes and presenting features in 85 consecutive patients with hypersensitivity pneumonitis. Mayo Clin Proc. 2007;82:812–6.
46. Barnes H, Lu J, Glaspole I, Collard HR, Johannson KA. Exposures and associations with clinical phenotypes in hypersensitivity pneumonitis: a scoping review. Respir Med. 2021;184:106444.
47. Barber CM, Wiggans RE, Carder M, Agius R. Epidemiology of occupational hypersensitivity pneumonitis; reports from the SWORD scheme in the UK from 1996 to 2015. Occup Environ Med. 2017;74:528–30.
48. Malmberg P, Rask-Andersen A, Höglund S, Kolmodin-Hedman B, Read GJ. Incidence of organic dust toxic syndrome and allergic alveolitis in Swedish farmers. Int Arch Allergy Appl Immunol. 1988;87:47–54.

49. Terho EO, Heinonen OP, Lammi S. Incidence of farmer's lung leading to hospitalization and its relation to meteorological observations in Finland. Acta Med Scand. 1983;213:295–8.
50. Huuskonen MS, Husman K, Järvisalo J, Korhonen O, Kotimaa M, Kuusela T, Nordman H, Zitting A, Mäntyjärvi R. Extrinsic allergic alveolitis in the tobacco industry. Br J Ind Med. 1984;41:77–83.
51. Orriols R, Aliaga JL, Antó JM, Ferrer A, Hernandez A, Rodrigo MJ, Morell F. High prevalence of mollusc shell hypersensitivity pneumonitis in nacre factory workers. Eur Respir J. 1997;10:780–6.
52. Vandenplas O, Malo JL, Dugas M, Cartier A, Desjardins A, Lévesque J, Shaughnessy MA, Grammer LC. Hypersensitivity pneumonitis-like reaction among workers exposed to diphenylmethane [correction to piphenylmethane] diisocyanate (MDI). Am Rev Respir Dis. 1993;147:338–46.
53. Baur X. Hypersensitivity pneumonitis (extrinsic allergic alveolitis) induced by isocyanates. J Allergy Clin Immunol. 1995;95:1004–10.
54. Banaszak EF, Thiede WH, Fink JN. Hypersensitivity pneumonitis due to contamination of an air conditioner. N Engl J Med. 1970;283:271–6.
55. Rose CS, Martyny JW, Newman LS, Milton DK, King TE Jr, Beebe JL, McCammon JB, Hoffman RE, Kreiss K. "Lifeguard lung": endemic granulomatous pneumonitis in an indoor swimming pool. Am J Public Health. 1998;88:1795–800.
56. Burton CM, Crook B, Scaife H, Evans GS, Barber CM. Systematic review of respiratory outbreaks associated with exposure to water-based metalworking fluids. Ann Occup Hyg. 2012;56:374–88.
57. Dalphin JC, Debieuvre D, Pernet D, Maheu MF, Polio JC, Toson B, Dubiez A, Monnet E, Laplante JJ, Depierre A. Prevalence and risk factors for chronic bronchitis and farmer's lung in French dairy farmers. Br J Ind Med. 1993;50:941–4.
58. Stanford CF, Hall G, Chivers A, Martin B, Nicholls DP, Evans J. Farmer's lung in Northern Ireland. Br J Ind Med. 1990;47:314–6.
59. Terho EO, Vohlonen I, Husman K. Prevalence and incidence of chronic bronchitis and farmer's lung with respect to socioeconomic factors. Eur J Respir Dis Suppl. 1987;152:29–36.
60. Hoppin JA, Umbach DM, Kullman GJ, Henneberger PK, London SJ, Alavanja MC, Sandler DP. Pesticides and other agricultural factors associated with self-reported farmer's lung among farm residents in the Agricultural Health Study. Occup Environ Med. 2007;64:334–41.
61. Banham SW, McSharry C, Lynch PP, Boyd G. Relationships between avian exposure, humoral immune response, and pigeon breeders' disease among Scottish pigeon fanciers. Thorax. 1986;41:274–8.
62. Rodríguez de Castro F, Carrillo T, Castillo R, Blanco C, Díaz F, Cuevas M. Relationships between characteristics of exposure to pigeon antigens. Clinical manifestations and humoral immune response. Chest. 1993;103:1059–63.
63. Cramer C, Schlünssen V, Bendstrup E, Stokholm ZA, Vestergaard JM, Frydenberg M, Kolstad HA. Risk of hypersensitivity pneumonitis and interstitial lung diseases among pigeon breeders. Eur Respir J. 2016;48:818–25.
64. Selman M, Pardo A, King TE Jr. Hypersensitivity pneumonitis: insights in diagnosis and pathobiology. Am J Respir Crit Care Med. 2012;186:314–24.
65. Lacasse Y, Selman M, Costabel U, Dalphin JC, Ando M, Morell F, Erkinjuntti-Pekkanen R, Muller N, Colby TV, Schuyler M, Cormier Y. Clinical diagnosis of hypersensitivity pneumonitis. Am J Respir Crit Care Med. 2003;168:952–8.
66. Yokoyama A, Kondo K, Nakajima M, Matsushima T, Takahashi T, Nishimura M, Bando M, Sugiyama Y, Totani Y, Ishizaki T, Ichiyasu H, Suga M, Hamada H, Kohno N. Prognostic value of circulating KL-6 in idiopathic pulmonary fibrosis. Respirology. 2006;11:164–8.
67. Takahashi H, Shiratori M, Kanai A, Chiba H, Kuroki Y, Abe S. Monitoring markers of disease activity for interstitial lung diseases with serum surfactant proteins A and D. Respirology. 2006;11 Suppl:S51–4.
68. Okamoto T, Tsutsui T, Suhara K, Furusawa H, Miyazaki Y, Inase N. Seasonal variation of serum KL-6 and SP-D levels in bird-related hypersensitivity pneumonitis. Sarcoidosis Vasc Diffuse Lung Dis. 2015;31:364–7.

69. Ohnishi H, Miyamoto S, Kawase S, Kubota T, Yokoyama A. Seasonal variation of serum KL-6 concentrations is greater in patients with hypersensitivity pneumonitis. BMC Pulm Med. 2014;14:129.
70. Allen DH, Basten A, Williams GV, Woolcock AJ. Familial hypersensitivity pneumonitis. Am J Med. 1975;59:505–14.
71. Okamoto T, Miyazaki Y, Tomita M, Tamaoka M, Inase N. A familial history of pulmonary fibrosis in patients with chronic hypersensitivity pneumonitis. Respiration. 2013;85:384–90.
72. Terwiel M, Grutters JC, van Moorsel CHM. Clustering of lung diseases in the family of interstitial lung disease patients. BMC Pulm Med. 2022;22:134.
73. Ley B, Newton CA, Arnould I, Elicker BM, Henry TS, Vittinghoff E, Golden JA, Jones KD, Batra K, Torrealba J, Garcia CK, Wolters PJ. The MUC5B promoter polymorphism and telomere length in patients with chronic hypersensitivity pneumonitis: an observational cohort-control study. Lancet Respir Med. 2017;5:639–47.
74. Katayanagi S, Setoguchi Y, Kitagawa S, Okamoto T, Miyazaki Y. Alternative gene expression by TOLLIP variant is associated with lung function in chronic hypersensitivity pneumonitis. Chest. 2022;161:458–69.
75. Ley B, Torgerson DG, Oldham JM, Adegunsoye A, Liu S, Li J, Elicker BM, Henry TS, Golden JA, Jones KD, Dressen A, Yaspan BL, Arron JR, Noth I, Hoffmann TJ, Wolters PJ. Rare protein-altering telomere-related gene variants in patients with chronic hypersensitivity pneumonitis. Am J Respir Crit Care Med. 2019;200:1154–63.
76. Stiehm ER, Reed CE, Tooley WH. Pigeon breeder's lung in children. Pediatrics. 1967;39:904–15.
77. Mastrorilli C, Pecoraro L, Arasi S, Barni S, Caminiti L, Castagnoli R, Giovannini M, Liotti L, Mori F, Saretta F, Marseglia GL, Novembre E. Pediatric hypersensitivity pneumonitis: literature update and proposal of a diagnostic algorithm. Ital J Pediatr. 2022;48:51.
78. Fink JN, Ortega HG, Reynolds HY, Cormier YF, Fan LL, Franks TJ, Kreiss K, Kunkel S, Lynch D, Quirce S, Rose C, Schleimer RP, Schuyler MR, Selman M, Trout D, Yoshizawa Y. Needs and opportunities for research in hypersensitivity pneumonitis. Am J Respir Crit Care Med. 2005;171:792–8.
79. Venkatesh P, Wild L. Hypersensitivity pneumonitis in children: clinical features, diagnosis, and treatment. Paediatr Drugs. 2005;7:235–44.
80. Griese M, Irnstetter A, Hengst M, Burmester H, Nagel F, Ripper J, Feilcke M, Pawlita I, Gothe F, Kappler M, Schams A, Wesselak T, Rauch D, Wittmann T, Lohse P, Brasch F, Kröner C. Categorizing diffuse parenchymal lung disease in children. Orphanet J Rare Dis. 2015;10:122.
81. Buchvald F, Petersen BL, Damgaard K, Deterding R, Langston C, Fan LL, Deutsch GH, Dishop MK, Kristensen LA, Nielsen KG. Frequency, treatment, and functional outcome in children with hypersensitivity pneumonitis. Pediatr Pulmonol. 2011;46:1098–107.
82. Griese M, Haug M, Hartl D, Teusch V, Glöckner-Pagel J, Brasch F. Hypersensitivity pneumonitis: lessons for diagnosis and treatment of a rare entity in children. Orphanet J Rare Dis. 2013;8:121.
83. Griese M. Chronic interstitial lung disease in children. Eur Respir Rev. 2018;27:170100.
84. Casamento K, Laverty A, Wilsher M, Twiss J, Gabbay E, Glaspole I, Jaffe A. Assessing the feasibility of a web-based registry for multiple orphan lung diseases: the Australasian Registry Network for Orphan Lung Disease (ARNOLD) experience. Orphanet J Rare Dis. 2016;11:42.
85. Cardoso J, Carvalho I. The value of family history in the diagnosis of hypersensitivity pneumonitis in children. J Bras Pneumol. 2014;40:183–7.

Chapter 3
Immunopathogenesis in Allergic Reaction, Inflammation, and Fibrosis

What Is Pathogenesis on Imunology of HP?

Takashi Yamana

1 Antigen Recognition and Sensitization (Fig. 3.1)

When inhaled antigens reach bronchioles and alveoli, antigen-presenting cells (APCs) recognize them by pattern recognition receptors (PRRs). Among PRRs, Toll-like receptor (TLR)2, TLR4, TRL6, TRL9, nucleotide-binding oligomerization domain-like receptors (NODs), and dectin-1 are mainly involved in the development of HP [1–3]. The signals driven by PRRs accelerate antigen uptake, innate

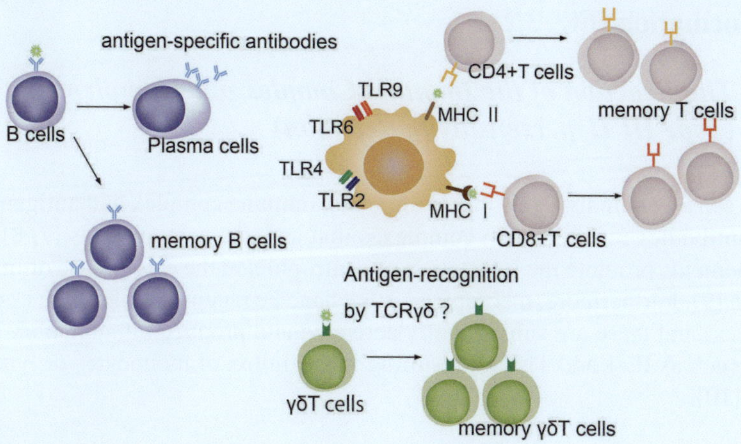

Fig. 3.1 The mechanism of antigen recognition and sensitization

T. Yamana (✉)
Department of Pulmonology, National Hospital Organization Disaster Medical Center, Tachikawa City, Japan

Y. Miyazaki (ed.), *Hypersensitivity Pneumonitis*, Respiratory Disease Series: Diagnostic Tools and Disease Managements,
https://doi.org/10.1007/978-981-96-7983-6_3

immune cells' activation, and production of inflammatory cytokines including IFN-g and IL-17A. After the recognition of antigens, APCs move to their regional lymph nodes or bronchus-associated lymphoid tissue (BALT) and present antigens to T cells by major histocompatibility complex (MHC), concurrently with the binding of costimulatory molecules to the ligands on T cells. In HP, APCs present antigens to CD4+ T cells by MHC classII and to CD8+ T cells by MHC classI [4]. Along with antigen presentation, APCs produce IL-12, which induces naïve T cells to differentiate into Th1 cells, and IL-1, and IL-23, which induce them to differentiate into Th17 cells. In addition, B cells recognize antigens and then differentiate into plasma cells that produce antigen-specific antibodies. Subsequently, these T and B cells persist as memory cells for a long period.

In addition to these mechanisms, a recent report revealed that γδ T cells play important roles in the sensitization of HP. γδ T cells are mainly distributed in mucosal tissues including skin, intestine, and lung and usually work as innate immune cells. However, γδ T cells are recently reported to work in recall responses just like traditional memory T cells in several murine bacteria-infection models and gathering attention as "memory γδ T cells." [5] Also in HP, the authors uncovered the pivotal role of memory γδ T cells using a murine HP model induced by pigeon-dropping extract (PDE) [6].

2 Infiltration of Inflammatory Cells and Granuloma Formation (Fig. 3.2)

2.1 *The Reaction of the Immune Complex and Complement (Type III Hypersensitivity Reaction)*

When sensitized individuals inhale antigens, immune complex and antigen-specific antibodies form immune complexes that activate complements [7, 8]. The complements promote the infiltration of neutrophils in the early phase of inflammation [9]. Furthermore, macrophages that have Fc receptors engulf the immune complex, and these are subsequently activated and produce inflammatory cytokines such as IL-1 and TNF-α, resulting in the influx of monocytes or lymphocytes [10].

2.2 *Granuloma Formation*

After the reaction of the immune complex and complements, inflammatory cells, including lymphocytes, monocytes, and macrophages, infiltrate the alveolar regions reached by the antigen. Th1 cytokines produced by T cells, IL-17A produced by γδ T cells, and various types of chemokines such as macrophage inflammatory

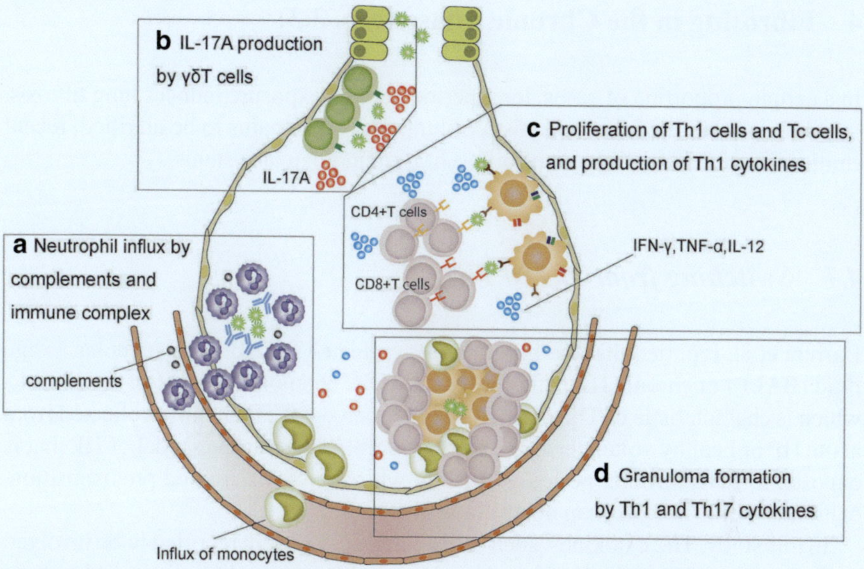

Fig. 3.2 The phase of infiltration of inflammatory cells and granuloma formation

protein-1 (MIP-1), monocyte chemoattractant protein-1 (MCP-1), interferon-gamma-induced protein 10 (IP-10), pulmonary and activation-regulated chemokine (PARC), and adhesion molecules, such as lymphocyte function-associated antigen-1 (LFA-1) and intercellular adhesion molecule 1 (ICAM-1), have important roles in this phase [6, 11–15]. Continuous antigen exposure results in prolonged infiltration of inflammatory cells, which leads to granuloma formation by clustered macrophages, monocytes, and lymphocytes [6].

3 Suppression of Pathogenesis by Regulatory T Cells

Regulatory T cells (Treg), which are one population of CD4+ T cells expressing FoxP3, suppress the immune response and induce immune tolerance by producing anti-inflammatory cytokines such as IL-10 or TGF-β, by suppression of antigen presentation, and by consumption of IL-2 [16]. Furthermore, FoxP3 inhibits the role of RorγT that works as a transcription factor in producing IL-17A by Th17 cells or γδ T cells [17]. Because FoxP3-deficient mice have been known for developing autoimmune diseases, Tregs are thought to be involved in many types of inflammatory or allergy diseases [18]. In the SR-induced mice model, Treg-deficient mice exhibited worse lung pathology than wild-type mice. In this study, Tregs were reported to impede the work of IFNγ-producing CD4+ cells and CD8+ cells [19]. Another study reported that Tregs collected from HP patients have weaker abilities to suppress activated T cells than those from healthy volunteers [20].

4 Fibrosing in the Chronic Phase (Fig. 3.3)

In a certain proportion of cases, long-period antigen exposure induces lung fibrosis.

Although the detailed mechanism of lung fibrosis remains to be clarified, recent studies report the involvement of different immunological systems.

4.1 *Switching from Th1 to Th2*

Barrera et al. reported that the lymphocytes collected from bronchoalveolar lavage fluid (BALF) of chronic HP patients express CXC chemokine receptor 4 (CXCR4), which is characteristic of Th2 cells, in a higher percentage than those collected from acute HP or healthy volunteers [21]. Furthermore, in the murine model of HP that is exposed to PDE for long period, A/J mice, which have Th2-biased predisposition, exhibited worse fibrosis than other kinds of mice [22].

In this study, Th2 cytokines, such as IL-4 and IL-13, were reported to be involved in the process of fibrosis. IL-13 is thought to induce the proliferation of fibrocytes directly or via TGF-β. A Th2-biased environment also induces epithelial–mesenchymal transition (EMT), which is said to be one of the mechanisms of fibrosis in different organs [23].

However, in the murine model of farmer's lung that is produced by the long-term administration of SR, not Th2 but Th17 cytokine is reported to have an important role in fibrosing of HP [24]. The precise mechanism of switching Th1 to Th2 is

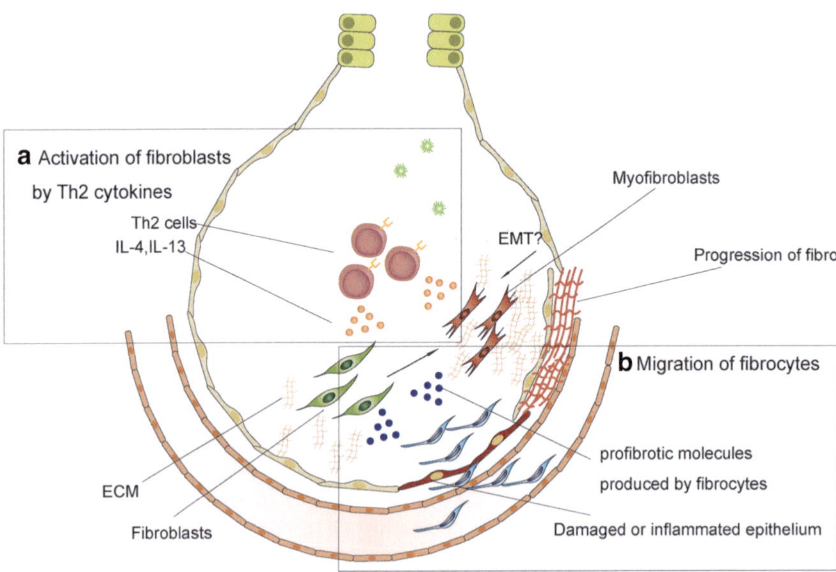

Fig. 3.3 Fibrosing in the chronic phase

poorly understood; therefore, further research is needed to uncover the role of Th2 and Th17 cytokines in the process of fibrosis in HP.

4.2 *Fibrocytes*

Fibrocytes, which are precursors of fibroblasts, are reported to be involved in the lung fibrosing of idiopathic lung fibrosis (IPF) [25]. Fibrocytes express leucocyte markers, for example, CD45, while they have characteristics of mesenchymal cells such as the production of collagen. They circulate in blood under steady states but have the ability to home to inflammatory sites [26]. A previous study reported that in chronic HP patients, fibrocytes increased in the lung and clustered in fibrosing areas by CXCR4 on fibrocytes and CXC chemokine ligand 12 (CXCL12) produced by epithelial cells. In this study, fibrocytes are thought to induce differentiation of fibroblasts into myofibroblasts, and to promote the production of collagen I and extracellular matrix (ECM) such as Matrix metalloproteinase-1 (MMP-1), resulting in lung fibrosis [27].

4.3 *Mucin Abnormalities*

Mucin is a glycoprotein that is contained in mucus and has crucial roles in defense against pathogens in mucous membranes. In a previous study, the existence of minor alleles of single nucleotide polymorphism (SNP) in MUC5B, which is one of the genes coding mucins, was shown to be a risk factor for IPF [28]. Similarly, a recent study reported that in HP patients, the existence of the minor alleles was related to the spreading of the fibrosing area [29]. Although the way how mucin abnormalities contribute to lung fibrosis is not clearly understood, a recent study using a bleomycin-induced murine model of lung fibrosis revealed that excessively produced Muc5b, which is coded by MUC5B, caused the decreased mucociliary clearance, resulting in lung fibrosis [30]. Another study reported that the mutant of MUC5B led to the overexpression of C3 and C3-deficient mice exhibited weaker lung fibrosis than the wild type, which implicated the relationship between C3 and lung fibrosis [31].

4.4 *γδ T Cells*

Whether γδ T cells, which were thought to work as accelerants in the inflammatory phase, contribute to fibrosis in HP is under discussion. In a previous study, γδ T cells were decreased in patients with fibrotic HP lung and were indicated to suppress lung fibrosis [32]. On the other hand, IL-17A produced by γδ T cells was reported to promote lung fibrosis in a murine model using SR. There are many types of γδ T cells that have different characters and roles: these can be, of course, distinguished by their unique signature surface markers and transcription factors. Therefore, further studies are needed to uncover what types of γδ T cells work in the inflammatory and fibrosing phases of HP.

References

1. Bhan U, Newstead MJ, Zeng X, et al. TLR9-dependent IL-23/IL-17 is required for the generation of Stachybotrys chartarum–induced hypersensitivity pneumonitis. J Immunol. 2013;190:349–56.
2. Fong DJ, Hogaboam CM, Matsuno Y. Toll-like receptor 6 drives interleukin-17A expression during experimental hypersensitivity pneumonitis. Immunology. 2010;130:125–36.
3. Higashino-Kameda M, Yabe-Wada T, Matsuba S, et al. A critical role of Dectin-1 in hypersensitivity pneumonitis. Inflamm Res. 2016;65:235–44.
4. Asakova M, Selman M, Morell F, Sterclova M, Molina-Molina M, Raghu G. Hypersensitivity pneumonitis: current concepts of pathogenesis and potential targets for treatment. Am J Respir Crit Care Med. 2019;200(3):301–8.
5. Khairallah C, Chu TH, Sheridan BS. Tissue adaptations of memory and tissue-resident gamma delta T cells. Front Immunol. 2018;9:2636.
6. Yamana T, Okamoto T, Ishizuka M. IL-17A-secreting memory γδ T cells play a pivotal role in sensitization and development of hypersensitivity pneumonitis. J Immunol. 2021;206(2):355–65.
7. Nielsen CH, Leslie RG. Complement's participation in acquired immunity. J Leukoc Biol. 2002;72:249–61.
8. Shanley T, Peters J, Jones M, et al. Reguratory effects of endogeneous interleukin-1 receptor antagonist protein in immunogloblin G immune complex-induecd lung injury. J Clin Invest. 1996;97:963.
9. Gao H, Neff T, Ward PA. Regulation of lung inflammation in the model of IgG immune-complex injury. Annu Rev Pathol. 1:215–42.
10. Haslam P, Dewar A, Butchers P, et al. Mast cells, atypical lymphocytes, and neutrophils in bronchoalveolar lavage in extrinsic allergic alveolitis. Comparison with other interstitial lung diseases. Am Rev Respir Dis. 1987;135:35–47.
11. Sugiyama Y, Kasahara T, Mukaida N, et al. Chemokine in bronchoalveolar lavage fluid in summer-type hypersensitivity pneumonitis. Eur Respir J. 1995;8:1084–90.
12. Fujimori Y, Kataoka M, Tada S, et al. The role of inteleukin-8 in interstitial pneumonia. Respirology. 2003;8:33–40.
13. Oshima M, Maeda A, Ishioka S, et al. Expression of C-C chemokine in bronochoalveolar lavage cells from patients with granulomatous lung diseases. Lung. 1999;177:229–40.
14. Kishi M, Miyazaki Y, Jinta T, et al. Pathogenesis of cBFL in common with IPF? Correlation of IP-10/TARC ratio with histological patterns. Thorax. 2008;63:810–6.
15. Pardo A, Smith KM, Abrams J, et al. CCL18/DC-CK-1/PARC up-regulation in hypersensitivity pneumonitis. J Leukoc Biol. 2001;70:610–6.
16. Palomares O, Martín-Fontecha M, Lauener R, et al. Regulatory T cells and immune regulation of allergic diseases: roles of IL-10 and TGF-β. Genes Immun. 2014;15(8):511–20.
17. Zhou L, Lopes JE, Chong MM, et al. TGF-beta-induced Foxp3 inhibits T(H)17 cell differentiation by antagonizing ROR-γt function. Nature. 2008;453(7192):236–40.
18. Hadaschik EN, Wei X, Leiss H, et al. Regulatory T cell-deficient scurfy mice develop systemic autoimmune features resembling lupus-like disease. Arthritis Res Ther. 2015;17(1):35.

19. Park Y, Oh SJ, Chung DH. CD4(+)CD25(+) regulatory T cells attenuate hypersensitivity pneumonitis by suppressing IFN-gamma production by CD4(+) and CD8(+) T cells. J Leukoc Biol. 2009;86:1427–37.
20. Girard M, Israël-Assayag E, Cormier Y. Impaired function of regulatory T-cells in hypersensitivity pneumonitis. Eur Respir J. 2011;37(3):632–9.
21. Barrera L, Mendoza F, Zuñiga J, et al. Functional diversity of T-cell subpopulations in subacute and chronic hypersensitivity pneumonitis. Am J Respir Crit Care Med. 2008;177(1):44.
22. Mitaka K, Miyazaki Y, Yasui M, Furuie M, Miyake S, Inase N, Yoshizawa Y. Th2-biased immune responses are important in a murine model of chronic hypersensitivity pneumonitis. Int Arch Allergy Immunol. 2011;154(3):264–74.
23. Yasui M, Miyazaki Y, Mitaka K, et al. Epithelial-mesenchymal transition in chronic hypersensitivity pneumonitis. J Med Dent Sci. 2012;59(1):29–41.
24. Andrews K, Ghosh MC, Schwingshackl A, et al. Chronic hypersensitivity pneumonitis caused by Saccharopolyspora rectivirgula is not associated with a switch to a Th2 response. Am J Physiol Lung Cell Mol Physiol. 2016;310(5):L393–402.
25. Moeller A, Gilpin SE, Ask K, et al. Circulating Fibrocytes are an indicator of poor prognosis in idiopathic pulmonary fibrosis. Am J Respir Crit Care Med. 2009;179:588–94.
26. Reilkoff RA, Bucala R, Herzog EL. Fibrocytes: emerging effector cells in chronic inflammation. Nat Rev Immunol. 2011;11:427–35.
27. García de Alba C, Buendia-Roldán I, Salgado A, et al. Fibrocytes contribute to inflammation and fibrosis in chronic hypersensitivity pneumonitis through paracrine effects. Am J Respir Crit Care Med. 2015;191(4):427–36.
28. Seibold MA, Wise AL, Speer MC, et al. A common MUC5B promoter polymorphism and pulmonary fibrosis. N Engl J Med. 2011;364(16):1503–12.
29. Furusawa H, Cardwell JH, Okamoto T, et al. Am J Respir Crit Care Med. 2020;202(10):1430–44.
30. Hancock LA, Hennessy CE, Solomon GM, et al. Muc5b overexpression causes mucociliary dysfunction and enhances lung fibrosis in mice. Nat Commun. 2018;9(1):5363. Published 2018 Dec 18
31. Okamoto T, Mathai SK, Hennessy CE, et al. The relationship between complement C3 expression and the MUC5B genotype in pulmonary fibrosis. Am J Physiol Lung Cell Mol Physiol. 2018;315(1):L1.
32. Simonian PL, Roark CL, Wehrmann F, et al. IL-17A-expressing T cells are essential for bacterial clearance in a murine model of hypersensitivity pneumonitis. J Immunol. 2009;182(10):6540–9.

Part II
Diagnosis

Chapter 4
Clinical Practice Guideline, ATS/JRS/ALAT2020, CHEST2021, JRS2022

What Are the Clinical Guidelines in HP?

Yoshikazu Inoue

1 Introduction

Hypersensitivity pneumonitis (HP) is typically an immune-mediated disease that manifests as interstitial lung disease (ILD) in susceptible individuals after exposure to an identified or unidentified factor [1, 2]. There was no official international standardized definition, diagnostic criteria, and diagnostic approach as of now despite efforts by international groups [1]. Walsh S et al. reported low levels of inter-multidisciplinary discussion team agreement for HP, which, for HP, might be in relation to the absence of evidence-based guidelines [3]. There were gaps of substantial regional frequencies about ILD, including HP [4]. Therefore, development of international clinical practice guideline was long awaited. Recently, two official guidelines, the official American Thoracic Society (ATS)/Japanese Respiratory Society (JRS)/ Asociacion Latinoamericana del Torax (ALAT) clinical practice guideline in 2020 [1] and the CHEST guideline and expert panel report in 2021, were published [5]. In addition, JRS published Japanese clinical practice guide 2022 in Japanese in 2022, and English version in 2024 [6]. Japanese guide was based on ATS.JRS/ALAT guideline, but added Japanese-specific issues and treatment and management of HP.

The purpose of this chapter is to introduce two official guidelines and one guide of HP, and to compare those guidelines and the guide.

Y. Inoue (✉)
Internal Medicine, Osaka Anti-tuberculosis Association, Osaka Fukujuji Hospital, Osaka, Japan

Clinical Research Center, NHO Kinki Chuo Chest Medical Center, Osaka, Japan

Y. Miyazaki (ed.), *Hypersensitivity Pneumonitis*, Respiratory Disease Series: Diagnostic Tools and Disease Managements,
https://doi.org/10.1007/978-981-96-7983-6_4

2 Diagnosis of HP in Adults. An Official ATS/JRS/ALAT Clinical Practice Guideline (ATS/JRS/ALAT 2020)

ATS/JRS/ALAT 2020 was the first international official guideline in the world for the diagnosis of HP published in 2020 [1]. Raghu G chaired and conducted an ad hoc subcommittee of the ATS, which was also endorsed by JRS and ALAT. A multidisciplinary (pulmonologists, radiologists, methodologists, pathologists, and patient) panel of experts from each discipline was constituted to identify clinically important questions related to diagnosis of HP among patients with newly identified ILD. The guideline was based on the National Academy of Medicine-adherent guideline methodology, including a full systematic review for each question and the formulation, writing, and grading of recommendations using the GRADE (Grading of Recommendations, Assessment, Development, and Evaluation) approach. This guideline consisted of definition, clinical manifestation, pathogenesis, radiological features, histopathological features, nonfibrotic or cellular HP and fibrotic HP, diagnostic criteria, diagnostic interventions including six clinical questions and recommendations, and future directions. Therapeutic clinical question or recommendation was not included [1].

2.1 *Definition of HP*

HP is defined as an inflammatory and/or fibrotic disease affecting the lung parenchyma and small airways. It typically results from an immune-mediated reaction provoked by an overt or occult inhaled antigen in susceptible individuals [1].

2.2 *Classification of HP*

HP was categorized into fibrotic HP (mixed inflammatory and fibrotic or purely fibrotic) or nonfibrotic HP, which were based on the predominant presence or absence of radiological and/or histopathological fibrosis. This new approach reflects the consensus that classification as fibrotic or nonfibrotic HP is more objective, and may reflect disease presentation, and is likely to be more consistently associated with the clinical course and other outcomes. Some patients may have mixed features; in such circumstances, the categorization is determined by the predominance of features [1].

2.3 *Natural History and Prognosis*

Patients with nonfibrotic HP who avoid ongoing exposure to the inciting agent may have a favorable prognosis with the possibility of stabilization or full recovery. Patients with fibrotic HP, particularly those with a usual interstitial pneumonia-like pattern, have reduced survival. Other features associated with poor prognosis include cigarette smoking, lower baseline vital capacity, lack of Bronchoalveolar lavage (BAL) lymphocytosis, persistent exposure to the inciting agent, and/or inability to identify an inciting agent. Notably, it has been reported that an inciting agent is not identified in 30–50% of cases evaluated at ILD referral centers [1].

2.4 Radiological Features of HP

Typical radiological features of HP (HRCT) include mosaic attenuation, air trapping, mosaic perfusion, and "three-density pattern." Based on chest HRCT scan features of HP, the nonfibrotic HP pattern was defined and classifieds into two HRCT patterns: typical HP, and compatible with HP (indeterminate for HP is not available). Chest HRCT scan features of the fibrotic HP Pattern were classified into three HRCT patterns: typical HP, compatible with HP, indeterminate for HP [1].

2.5 Histopathologic Features of HP

The nonfibrotic HP histopathologic pattern (cellular HP) was defined and classified into three histopathological patterns: HP, probable HP, indeterminate for HP. Fibrotic HP was defined and classified into three histopathological patterns: HP, probable HP, indeterminate for HP [1].

2.6 Diagnosis of HP

When a patient presents with newly detected ILD identified by HRCT, the clinician should be prompted to elicit a careful and thorough history and possibly utilize formal questionnaires to reveal the possibility of a temporal relationship between environmental factors/exposures and the onset of symptoms. Serum IgG antibody testing against potential antigens associated with HP may also be performed to detect exposure to potential inciting agents of HP. Many patients should proceed to BAL with lymphocyte cellular analysis with or without transbronchial lung biopsy, and if this information, accompanied by the HRCT patterns, is insufficient to make a definitive diagnosis, they should undergo an MDD followed by transbronchial lung biopsy, transbronchial lung cryo-biopsy, or surgical lung biopsy. This approach is recommended by experts in HP on the basis of the best available evidence. This approach should be reevaluated as and when new evidence crops in and should be modified as needed (Fig. 4.1). Figure 4.2 shows the algorithm for the diagnostic evaluation of possible HP.

HRCT	Typical for HP		Compatible with HP		Indeterminate for HP	
History of exposure and/or serum IgG testing	Exposure +	Exposure –	Exposure +	Exposure –	Exposure +	Exposure –
No BAL or BAL without lymphocytosis and either no histopathology or indeterminate histopathology	*Moderate confidence*	*Low confidence*	*Low confidence*	*Not Excluded*	*Not Excluded*	*Not Excluded*
BAL lymphocytosis without histopathology sampling	*High confidence*	*Moderate confidence*	*Moderate confidence*	*Low confidence*	*Low confidence*	*Not Excluded*
BAL lymphocytosis with indeterminate histopathology	*Definite*	*High confidence*	*Moderate confidence*	*Moderate confidence*	*Low confidence*	*Not Excluded*
Probable HP histopathology	*Definite*	*High confidence*	*High confidence*	*Moderate confidence*	*Moderate confidence*	*Low confidence*
Typical HP histopathology	*Definite*	*Definite*	*Definite*	*Definite*	*Definite*	*High confidence**

Fig. 4.1 HP diagnosis based on incorporation of imaging, exposure assessment, BAL lymphocytosis, and histopathological findings (ATS/JRS/ALAT 2020) (Modified from Ref. [1]). All confidence levels are subject to multidisciplinary discussion. *Confidence may increase to "definite" if the pathologist's conclusion persists after reevaluation in the context of additional clinical information or an expert's second opinion on histopathology. We categorized diagnoses as definite (≧90% confidence), high-confidence, (80–89%), moderate-confidence (70–79%), and low-confidence (51–69%) diagnoses. HP hypersensitivity pneumonitis, HRCT high-resolution computed tomography

2.7 Confidence Levels of the Diagnosis

According to the confidence levels evaluated by combination of HRCT pattern, history of exposure and/or serum IgG testing, BAL lymphocytosis, and histopathology pattern, the diagnosis was categorized into five (Fig. 4.1): "Definite" (≧90% confidence), "High confidence" (80–89%), "Moderate confidence" (70–79%), "Low confidence" (51–69%), and "Not excluded." Confidence levels are defined as previously described [7]. All confidence levels are subject to multidisciplinary discussion (MDD) [1].

2.8 Clinical Questions and Recommendations

Six clinical questions about the diagnosis of HP were listed, and after the systematic review of each question, voting by the committee members were performed to determine recommendation and evidence levels (Table 4.1) [1].

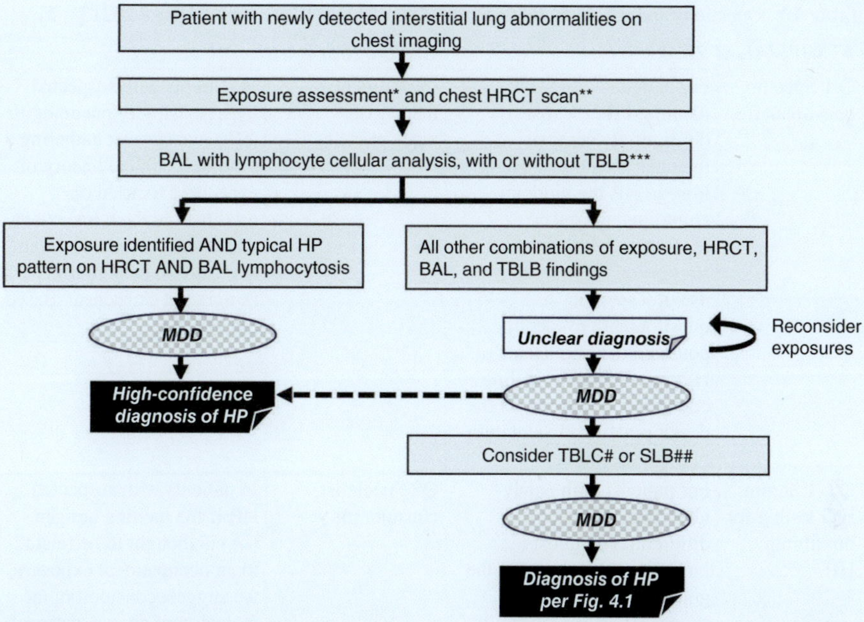

Fig. 4.2 Algorithm for the diagnostic evaluation of possible HP (ATS/JRS/ALAT 2020) (Modified from Ref. [1]). Specific features are described for all steps of the algorithm in the corresponding sections of the manuscript. A provisional diagnosis may be adequate in patients for whom the differential diagnosis has been sufficiently narrowed such that further investigations are unlikely to alter management, when invasive testing has unacceptable risks, or when such tests are declined by the patient. *Exposure assessment includes a thorough clinical history and/or serum IgG testing against potential antigens associated with HP and/or, in centers with the appropriate expertise and experience, specific inhalational challenge testing. **High-resolution computed tomography should be performed using the technique described in CHEST 2021 and then reviewed with a thoracic radiologist. ***Transbronchial lung biopsy is suggested for patients with potential nonfibrotic HP. #TBLC is suggested for patients with potential nonfibrotic HP, depending on local expertise. ##SLB is infrequently considered in patients with nonfibrotic HP. HRCT high-resolution computed tomography, SLB surgical lung biopsy, TBLB transbronchial lung biopsy, TBLC transbronchial lung cryobiopsy

Table 4.1 Questions and recommendations of ATS/JRS/ALAT 2020 and CHEST 2021 [1, 5]

ATS/JRS/ALAT 2020		CHEST 2021	
Q 1 Specific questionnaire	For patients with newly identified ILD whose differential diagnosis includes nonfibrotic HP or fibrotic HP, the guideline committee makes no recommendation or suggestion for or against the use of a specific questionnaire to identify potential inciting agents of HP; instead, the guideline committee recommends the development and validation of a questionnaire.	Q1 Clinical history of exposures	In patients with suspected hypersensitivity pneumonitis (HP), we suggest gathering a thorough clinical history of exposures focused on establishing the type, extent, and temporal relationship of exposure(s) to symptoms (Ungraded Consensus-Based Statement).
Q2–1 Serum IgG testing for nonfibrotic HP	For patients with newly identified ILD whose differential diagnosis includes nonfibrotic HP, the guideline committee suggests performing serum IgG testing that targets potential antigens associated with HP (suggestion, very low confidence in the estimated effects).	Q2 Specialist consultation	In patients with suspected HP, if the inciting antigen (IA) is thought to be related to an occupational exposure, we suggest considering the inclusion of an occupational medicine specialist and an environmental hygienist during the multidisciplinary diagnostic workup, especially when the source of exposure is obscure or unverified (Ungraded Consensus-Based Statement).
Q2–2 Serum IgG testing for fibrotic HP	For patients with newly identified ILD whose differential diagnosis includes fibrotic HP, the guideline committee suggests performing serum IgG testing that targets potential antigens associated with HP (suggestion, very low confidence in the estimated effects).	Q3 Identification of inciting antigens	In patients with suspected HP, we suggest classifying patients based on the likelihood of an occupational or environmental inciting antigen exposure (Weak Recommendation, Very Low-Quality Evidence).

(continued)

Table 4.1 (continued)

ATS/JRS/ALAT 2020		CHEST 2021	
Q3–1 BAL for nonfibrotic HP	For patients with newly identified ILD whose differential diagnosis includes nonfibrotic HP, the guideline committee recommends BAL with lymphocyte cellular analysis (recommendation, very low confidence in the estimated effects).	Q4 Classification of HP	For patients with either newly diagnosed or a working diagnosis of HP, we suggest classifying the disease as fibrotic or nonfibrotic based on the presence or absence of fibrosis on high-resolution CT (HRCT) of the chest (Weak Recommendation, Very Low-Quality Evidence).
Q3–2 BAL for fibrotic HP	For patients with newly identified ILD whose differential diagnosis includes fibrotic HP, the guideline committee suggests BAL with lymphocyte cellular analysis (suggestion, very low confidence in the estimated effects).	Q5 Clinical improvement with antigen avoidance	In patients with suspected HP, if an IA exposure is identified and then completely avoided, we suggest using clinical improvement with antigen avoidance to support the diagnosis of HP, but not relying solely on the lack of clinical improvement with antigen avoidance to rule out the diagnosis of HP (Weak Recommendation, Very Low-Quality Evidence).
Q4–1 TBBx for nonfibrotic HP	For patients with newly identified ILD whose differential diagnosis includes nonfibrotic HP, the guideline committee suggests TBBx (suggestion, very low confidence in the estimated effects).	Q6 Clinical improvement with medical therapy.	For patients with suspected HP, we suggest not relying solely on clinical improvement with medical therapy to confirm a diagnosis of HP or on the lack of clinical improvement with medical therapy alone to rule out the diagnosis of HP (Weak Recommendation, Very Low-Quality Evidence).
Q4–2 TBBx for fibrotic HP	For patients with newly identified ILD whose differential diagnosis includes fibrotic HP, the guideline committee makes no recommendation or suggestion for or against TBBx.	Q7 Antigen-specific antibody testing.	For patients with suspected HP, we suggest not relying solely on serum antigen-specific immunoglobulin G (IgG) or immunoglobulin A (IgA) testing to confirm or rule out the diagnosis of HP (Weak Recommendation, Very Low-Quality Evidence).

(continued)

Table 4.1 (continued)

ATS/JRS/ALAT 2020		CHEST 2021	
Q5–1 TBLC for nonfibrotic HP	For patients with newly identified ILD whose differential diagnosis includes nonfibrotic HP, the guideline committee makes no recommendation or suggestion for or against TBLC.	Q8 Antigen-specific inhalation challenge testing.	For patients with suspected HP, we suggest not performing antigen-specific inhalation challenge testing to support the diagnosis of HP (Weak Recommendation, Very Low-Quality Evidence).
Q5–2 TBLC for fibrotic HP	For patients with newly identified ILD whose differential diagnosis includes fibrotic HP, the guideline committee suggests TBLC (suggestion, very low confidence in estimated effects).	Q9 Specific lymphocyte proliferation testing	For patients with suspected HP, we suggest not performing antigen-specific lymphocyte proliferation testing to support the diagnosis of HP (Weak Recommendation, Very Low-Quality Evidence).
Q6–1 SLB for nonfibrotic HP	For patients with newly identified ILD whose differential diagnosis includes nonfibrotic HP, the guideline committee suggests SLB; this recommendation is intended for after alternative diagnostic options have been exhausted (suggestion, very low confidence in estimated effects).	Q10 High-resolution CT pattern	For patients with suspected HP, we suggest the integration of HRCT findings characteristic of HP with clinical findings to support the diagnosis of HP, but not using the CT findings in isolation to make a definite diagnosis (Weak Recommendation, Very Low-Quality Evidence).
Q6–2 SLB for fibrotic HP	For patients with newly identified ILD whose differential diagnosis includes fibrotic HP, the guideline committee suggests SLB; this recommendation is intended for after alternative diagnostic options have been exhausted (suggestion, very low confidence in estimated effects).	Q11 Multidisciplinary discussion	For patients with suspected HP, we suggest using a multidisciplinary discussion (MDD) for diagnostic decision making (Weak Recommendation, Very Low- Quality Evidence).

(continued)

Table 4.1 (continued)

ATS/JRS/ALAT 2020		CHEST 2021	
		Q12 BAL cellular analysis.	For patients with suspected HP who have a compelling exposure history within the appropriate clinical context and a chest HRCT pattern typical for HP, we suggest not routinely using BAL fluid analysis to confirm a diagnosis of HP (Weak Recommendation, Very Low-Quality Evidence).
		Q13 Lung biopsy	In patients with suspected HP, we suggest considering histological lung biopsy for additional diagnostic evaluation when all available data such as clinical, laboratory, and radiologic findings along with bronchoscopic results do not yield a confident diagnosis and results may help guide management (Weak Recommendation, Very Low-Quality Evidence).
		Q14 Lung biopsy pattern	For patients with suspected HP, we suggest integrating biopsy findings with clinical and radiological findings to support the diagnosis of HP in the context of the MDD (Weak Recommendation, Very Low-Quality Evidence).

3 Diagnosis and Evaluation of Hypersensitivity Pneumonitis CHEST Guideline and Expert Panel Report (CHEST 2021)

In 2021, Pérez ERF et al. published CHEST 2021, as a chair by the evaluation by CHEST's Professional Standards Committee. The international panel consisted of the guideline chair, 13 panelists, representing seven countries, a methodologist, and an additional panelist serving as a liaison to CHEST's Guidelines Oversight Committee. This multidisciplinary panel includes experts in ILDs, occupational and environmental medicine, chest radiology, and pulmonary pathology [5].

While ATS/JRS/ALAT 2020 shared similar aims, CHEST 2021 addressed a number of key diagnostic questions not covered in ATS/JRS/ALAT 2020 and thus reviewed and analyzed an additional comprehensive body of corresponding evidence [5].

3.1 Definition of HP

HP is an immunologically mediated form of lung disease resulting from inhalational exposure to a large variety of environmental and/or occupational organic (typically fungal, bacterial, and avian), and less often, nonorganic inciting antigens (IAs). HP is a complex lung disease that occurs in genetically susceptible individuals previously sensitized to the inhaled IA [5].

3.2 Radiological Features of HP

HRCT categories of nonfibrotic HP patterns were classified into two patterns: Typical nonfibrotic HP and Compatible with nonfibrotic HP. HRCT categories of fibrotic HP patterns were classified into three patterns: typical fibrotic HP, compatible with fibrotic HP, indeterminate for fibrotic HP [5].

3.3 Histopathologic Features (If Appropriate) of HP

Histologic diagnostic criteria for nonfibrotic HP pattern are classified into four patterns: typical nonfibrotic HP, compatible with nonfibrotic HP, indeterminate for nonfibrotic HP, alternative diagnosis [5].

3.4 Diagnosis of HP

Figure 4.3 shows the algorithm for the diagnosis of fibrotic and nonfibrotic hypersensitivity pneumonitis [5].

Despite conceptual and organizational differences in the HRCT images and histopathological pattern description in ATS/JRS/ALAT 2020, diagnostic approaches of ATS/JRS/ALAT 2020 and CHEST 2021 guidelines share several similarities. Important differences between CHEST2021 and the guidance provided by ATS/JRS/ALAT 2020 regarding IA characterization (e.g., establishing the IA likelihood vs. dichotomizing the exposure into "yes" or "no"), the use of a structured questionnaire to optimize exposure identification and pretest likelihood, when to perform

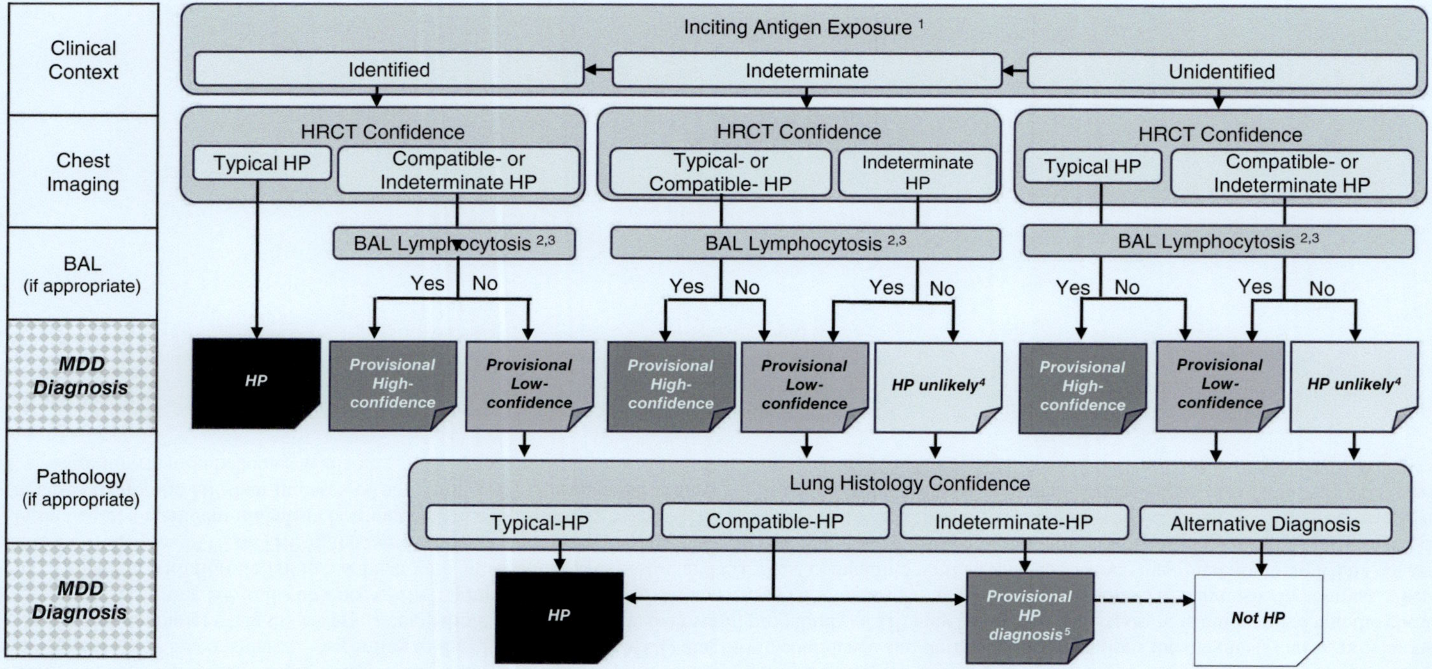

Fig. 4.3 Algorithm for the diagnosis of fibrotic and nonfibrotic HP (CHEST 2021) (Modified from Ref. [5]). *The diagnostic confidences are not intended to represent arbitrary estimates of the probability of HP diagnosis before and after testing but rather to provide a conceptual model for assessing discordant information and help optimize diagnostic clinical reasoning when evaluating patients with suspected HP. HRCT high-resolution CT, MDD multidisciplinary discussion. [1]The certainty of the IA cause and source may change over time after reevaluating additional exposure and clinical data. When the inciting antigen exposure is indeterminate or unidentified, alternative nonfibrotic causes commonly not captured by history include primary bronchiolar disorders. A detailed history may help identify infections, recurrent

Fig. 4.3 (continued) aspiration, pneumoconiosis, other granulomatous lung diseases, smoking- or immunodeficiency-related ILD, drug/dust inhalation, and connective tissue disorders. [2]The BAL in this algorithm does not imply that every suspected HP case needs to undergo this test. Instead, the objective is to show the estimated level of diagnostic confidence when the BAL fluid analysis results are combined with the clinical context and chest imaging confidence level. BAL lymphocytosis (eg. $\geqq$20%) alone may not rule out HP but should be interpreted in by taking into account the entire cellular count differential, sampling site, and protocol as well as the clinical context including age, smoking history, and treatment. A marked increase in BAL lymphocyte percentage is of additional value in distinguishing HP from other forms of interstitial lung disease (ILD). While in fibrotic HP, the absence of BAL fluid lymphocytosis does not rule out the disease and the level of uncertainty generally remains unchanged, in nonfibrotic HP, the level of confidence is substantially reduced, especially when the IA exposure is indeterminate or unidentified. Cutoffs that define abnormal increases in BAL lymphocyte counts to accurately distinguish HP from other ILDs remain to be determined. [3]Until further evidence becomes available, transbronchial biopsies may be considered. [4]According to the clinical context, MDD diagnostic confidence and during serial evaluations the diagnosis can be provisional or ultimately HP. For example, when the biopsy is compatible with fibrotic HP, the overall probability of HP may be lower if the exposure is unidentified and the chest CT is indeterminate for fibrotic HP in the absence of BAL lymphocytosis. The MDD consensus HP diagnosis may lead to a provisional HP diagnosis. In contrast, when the biopsy is compatible with fibrotic HP in a subject with an identifiable exposure and CT chest compatible with HP, the confidence may increase to an MDD consensus HP diagnosis. If the pre-VATS or TBC diagnosis confidence is unlikely for HP, a biopsy showing typical histopathology for HP may lead to an MDD provisional diagnosis. In this case, a confident diagnosis is sometimes made, especially when MDD prompts review and revision of the initial clinical context. [5]This scenario is more likely in cases of fibrotic HP than in cases of nonfibrotic HP. During serial multidisciplinary discussion evaluations, the diagnosis may change to "not HP" (dashed arrow), as more information becomes available

serum-antigen-specific antibody testing, specific inhalational challenge testing, and the determination of HP diagnostic confidence. Another important difference is when to pursue BAL fluid analysis. The guideline committee does not recommend BAL with lymphocyte cellular analysis in all subjects, particularly in those with a compelling exposure history within the appropriate clinical context and a chest HRCT pattern typical for HP. In high prevalence settings, such as nonfibrotic HP, such a combination may be sufficiently predictive of histopathological HP to forgo BAL (or lung biopsy). BAL fluid analysis should be considered to evaluate for an additional reason according to the pretest estimate and/or if the pretest probability of HP is in the middle, above the test threshold and below the treatment threshold [5].

In CHEST 2021, first, the diagnostic approach to HP is step-wise, patient centered, and ideally based on multidisciplinary evaluation. Second, while nonfibrotic HP cases with an identified IA may be solved by pattern recognition, complex cases including those with fibrotic HP may require a hypothetico-deductive diagnostic approach [5].

Third, this diagnostic approach integrates the steps above into the multidisciplinary assessment to help establish the level of diagnostic confidence before determining the need for further testing during the HP diagnostic process.

Fourth, the diagnostic approach to HP is guided by the degree of diagnostic certainty required. Patients without a confident diagnosis but in whom HP is suspected have a provisional diagnosis underscoring the importance of reviewing the diagnosis (e.g., an indeterminate IA) at regular intervals. That the provisional diagnosis might change highlights the value of seeking additional expertise or multidisciplinary team consultation to help confirm or reject the working diagnosis. The diagnostic process is iterative and should be revisited as additional data become available.

Fifth, this diagnostic approach uses the terms: high or low confidence. The ultimate goal of classification of a provisional diagnosis as high or low confidence is to prevent inappropriate testing, such as overutilization of TBC or VATS for diagnosis verification, in patients with a provisional high confidence diagnosis. However, in some cases, diagnostic uncertainty remains, even after VATS or TBC, preventing a clear differentiation of HP from an unclassifiable ILD. In this scenario, in the absence of a predominant alternative cause, the term "provisional" is used.

Sixth, the diagnostic algorithm does not supersede clinical judgment regarding when to stop diagnostic investigations and start treatment or the impact of disease behavior on informing test-treatment thresholds. For example, despite the importance of identifying and abating an IA, a timely and accurate diagnosis might not be possible or necessary in all fibrotic HP subjects with a progressive phenotype for treatment to be justified in the context of MDD consensus.

Finally, the presented imaging and histopathological categories and the diagnostic approach do not capture each and every HP case. These should be viewed as conditional and will evolve as new evidence becomes available [5].

3.5 Confidence Category of HP Diagnosis

CHEST 2021 presents a 4 four-tiered ontology: HP: Confident diagnosis (≧90%), Provisional high- confidence (70–89%), Provisional Low-confidence; (51–69%), HP Unlikely (<50%) (Table 4.2) [5, 7].

3.6 Clinical Questions and Recommendations

The expert panel drafted 14 key clinical questions using the Population, Intervention, Comparator, Outcome (PICO) format. The methodologist performed an initial systematic search of the literature for all PICO questions in March 2018. A pragmatic search update was conducted in May 2020 to identify relevant studies published after the original literature search. The recommendations to the 14 questions are listed in Table 4.1 [5].

Table 4.2 Comparison of ATS/JRS/ALAT 2020, CHEST 2021, and JRS 2022 [1, 5, 6]

	ATS/JRS/ALAT 2020	CHEST 2021	JRS 2022
Guideline or guide	Guideline	Guideline	Guide
Publication	Am J Respir Crit Care Med in 2020	Chest in 2021	Book in 2024 (Katsuseido, JRS, Japanese version) Respir Investig in 2024 (English version)
Language	English	English	Japanese and English
Endorsed Society	ATS, JRS, ALAT	ACCP	JRS
Review	Systematic review	Systematic review	Narrative review
Evaluation of recommendation, evidence	GRADE	CHEST grading system	No
Clinical questions	6 questions	14 questions	No
Classification of HP	Nonfibrotic HP Fibrotic HP	Nonfibrotic HP Fibrotic HP	Nonfibrotic HP Fibrotic HP (acute, chronic, etc., were mentioned)
Diagnosis	Yes	Yes	Yes
Clinical context	Exposure assessment (history of exposure and/or serum IgG testing etc.,)	Exposure assessment (inciting antigen, identified/indeterminate/unidentified, etc.,)	Japanese-specific serum IgG, antigen identification, other serum biomarkers, etc., Japan-specific modifications

(continued)

Table 4.2 (continued)

	ATS/JRS/ALAT 2020	CHEST 2021	JRS 2022
Guideline or guide	Guideline	Guideline	Guide
HRCT imaging	2 patterns for nonfibrotic HP, and 3 patterns for fibrotic HP	2 patterns for nonfibrotic HP, and 3 patterns for fibrotic HP	Basically ATS/JRS/ALAT 2020 with modification
BAL	Yes	Yes	Yes
Pathology	3 patterns for nonfibrotic HP, and 3 patterns for fibrotic HP	4 patterns for nonfibrotic HP, and 4 patterns for fibrotic HP	Basically ATS/JRS/ALAT 2020
Confidence level of diagnostic categories	5 categories Definite (≧90%), High confidence (80–89%), Moderate confidence (70–79%), Low confidence (51–69%), Not excluded (<50%).	4 categories HP: Confident diagnosis (≧90%), Provisional high confidence (70–89%). Provisional low confidence (51–69%). HP Unlikely (<50%).	Basically ATS/JRS/ALAT 2020
MDD	Yes	Yes	Yes
Treatment	No	No	Yes

4 Japanese Clinical Practice Guide 2022 for HP (JRS 2022)

After the publications of two official guidelines for the diagnosis of HP, JRS published its own Japanese clinical practice guide for HP. JRS officially endorsed the ATS/JRS/ALAT 2020 guideline, but JRS needs to add several Japan-specific issues of HP. Tomioka H and Miyazaki Y organized the JRS official guide committee as cochairs with the support of The Japanese Society of Allergology, The Japanese Society of Occupational and Environmental Allergy, The Japan Society of Sarcoidosis and Other Granulomatous Disorders, and the Survey and Research grants from the Ministry of Health, Labour and Welfare, the Study Group on Diffuse Pulmonary Disorders, and Scientific Research/Research on Intractable Diseases for cooperation.

The heterogeneity in disease forms and overlapping presentations with other types of ILD further add to the diagnostic challenge. A diagnosis of HP should therefore be considered in any patient presenting with ILD, and a thorough review of potential exposures is necessary [6].

4.1 Definition

JRS 2022 defined that HP was an allergic or immune disease that occurs when repeated inhalation of antigens leads to inflammation, mainly characterized by lymphocyte infiltration of the alveolar septa and bronchioles, and it typically results from an immune-mediated reaction provoked by an overt or occult inhaled antigen in susceptible individuals, which was compatible with the ATS/JRS/ALAT 2020 [1, 6].

4.2 Classification

In Japan, HP was historically classified into acute, subacute, and chronic HP. However, cluster analysis using clinical variables has demonstrated that it can also be appropriately classified into acute and chronic HP, and Yoshizawa et al. and Ohtani et al. [1] further subclassified chronic HP into insidious and recurrent types, respectively (Fig. 4.4) [6].

In some cases of the recurrent type, acute symptoms, such as fever, are relieved between relapses; however, dyspnea is known to gradually develop with the progression of pulmonary fibrosis. ATS/JRS/ALAT 2020 opted not to adopt the acute/subacute/chronic classifications and decided nonfibrotic and fibrotic classifications, because fibrotic changes were prognostic. The designation cellular HP was also listed as a histopathological classification of nonfibrotic HP [1]. Several reports demonstrate that the nonfibrotic and fibrotic classification offers a better reflection of disease progression and prognosis than the acute, subacute, and chronic classification. By merging both classifications, it becomes evident that all cases of acute HP are nonfibrotic, while chronic HP can be either nonfibrotic or fibrotic. Consequently, HP can be categorized into three types: acute HP, chronic nonfibrotic

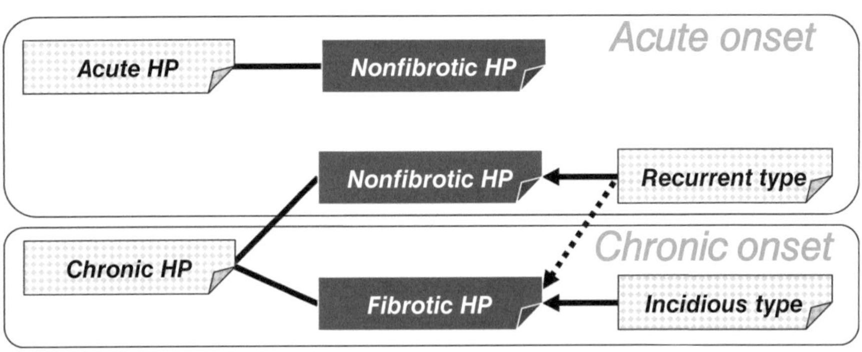

Fig. 4.4 Clinical entity form of HP. (JRS 2022) (Modified from Ref. [6]). ※ In some cases of the recurrent type, acute symptoms, such as fever, are relieved between relapses; however, dyspnea is known to gradually develop as pulmonary fibrosis progresses

HP, and chronic fibrotic HP. Chronic nonfibrotic HP corresponds to the recurrent type, whereas chronic fibrotic HP corresponds to the insidious type. JRS 2022 guide basically uses the classification of ATS/JRS/ALAT 2020. However, JRS 2022 noted that the term acute HP is consistent with the concept that has been used [6].

4.3 Major Types of HP in Japan

Major types of HP in Japan include summer type, home related, bird related, farmer's lung, painter's lung, humidifier lung, and mushroom grower's lung. Identifying causative antigens is critical for increasing diagnostic confidence, as well as improving prognosis through appropriate antigen avoidance. JRS 2022 proposes a comprehensive antigen questionnaire including the outbreak sources reported in Japan [6, 8].

4.4 Diagnosis of HP

The specific details of the diagnostic criteria in ATS/JRS/ALAT 2020, regarding the diagnostic algorithm (Fig. 4.2), were omitted. However, the following four annotations were written by the committee organized by the JRS to facilitate the interpretation of the content and correlate the medical situation in Japan [6].

- Clinical practice guide annotation #1: checking biomarkers.
  The measurement of KL-6 is recommended for "patients newly identified with an abnormal interstitial shadow on chest imaging." Seasonal changes in the KL-6 concentration (increase in winter for bird related HP/humidifier lung and in summer for summer-type HP) and high KL-6 concentrations provide a basis for the suspicion of HP [6, 9].
- Clinical practice guide annotation #2: measurement of serum-specific IgG.
  In Japan, medical insurance covers the assessments of bird-specific IgG (pigeons, budgerigars) and the *T. asahii* antibody [6, 10].
- Clinical practice guide annotation #3: antigen exposure assessment (exposure assessment).
  The 2021 CHEST guideline recommends continuous detailed medical history taking and classifying patients based on three designations (identified, indeterminate, and unidentified) for the identification of the causative antigen. If the causative antigen is identified, the capacity to avoid the causative antigen during each medical examination should be confirmed. If the causative antigen has not been identified, environmental surveys and the environmental provocation test at home and the workplace should also be considered. In Fig. 4.2 of ATS/JRS/ALAT 2020, the confidence level is considered as "Definite" if both the radiological (HRCT) and pathological findings are typical for HP. However, even in these cases, it is important to specify and avoid the causative antigen [6].

- Clinical practice guide annotation #4: fibrotic HRCT pattern.
  Basically, the same classification of ATS/JRS/ALAT 2020 is followed here too. The fibrotic HRCT pattern of ATS/JRS/ALAT 2020 was reviewed by this committee and revised for easier understanding [6].

4.5 *Treatments*

Antigen avoidance is critical for disease management of HP. JRS 2022 also addresses the pharmacological management of HP, highlighting the treatment strategy for fibrotic HP including combination therapies with anti-inflammatory/immunosuppressive and antifibrotic drugs [6].

Please see the section of treatment in detail.

5 Integrated Approach of Fibrotic HP and Idiopathic Pulmonary Fibrosis

In 2018, the clinical practice guidelines for the diagnosis of idiopathic pulmonary fibrosis (IPF) were published and in 2022 [11, 12], the guideline was updated by ATS/ERS/JRS/ALAT. Now, the HP guideline was published. These disease-specific guidelines were developed independently, without clear direction on how to apply their respective recommendations concurrently within a single patient, where discrimination between these two fibrotic interstitial lung diseases represents a frequent diagnostic challenge. Marinescu DC et al. published a pragmatic approach on how to apply existing guidelines to distinguish IPF and fHP and proposed algorithms to integrate two guidelines of HP and IPF [13]. Marinescu DC et al. applied the Integrated Approach to the Canadian Registry for Pulmonary Fibrosis, and concluded that an integrated approach to guideline-defined UIP and fHP patterns is feasible and supports >5% gas trapping as an important criterion. Typical or probable UIP and typical fHP patterns have moderate predictive values for a corresponding diagnosis of IPF and fHP, although occasionally confounded by CTD-ILD; compatible fHP is nonspecific [14, 15].

6 Comparison of Two Clinical Practice Guidelines

The two guidelines present differing algorithmic approaches to arrive at a confident diagnosis, with strong considerations of diagnostic likelihood. Both guidelines present criteria for establishing the diagnosis in a patient with ILD suspected to have HP, with a few differences, using combinations of several specific features to support or rule out disease.

Basically, same classification of ATS/JRS/ALAT 2020 presents five grades of confidence: definite (0.90% diagnostic likelihood), high confidence (80–89%), moderate confidence (70–79%), low confidence (51–69%), and HP considered but not excluded (<50%). CHEST 2021 presents a four-tiered ontology: confident diagnosis (0.90%), provisional high confidence (70–89%), provisional low confidence (51–69%), and unlikely (<50%, as previously proposed).

Buendía-Roldán I et al. applied the diagnostic criteria of two guidelines to 144 cases with a previously confirmed diagnosis of HP [16]. They found Definite = 18%, High confidence = 42%, Moderate confidence = 34%, Low confidence = 4%, Not excluded = 2% by ATS/JRS/ALAT 2020, and HP = 65%, Provisional high-confidence = 27%, Provisional low-confidence = 7%, HP Unlikely = 1% [1, 5, 13].

Although, there are limitations to their study, despite the fact that both guidelines use similar domains for the diagnosis of HP, the agreement between them was low for the definitive/high-confidence diagnosis among patients included in this study. The questions remain as to whether we are going to overdiagnose HP with the CHEST algorithm (patient's respiratory problem is mistakenly attributed to HP when another ILD is responsible) or underdiagnose HP by applying the ATS/JRS/ALAT algorithm. In either situation, the inaccurate identification of fibrotic HP, instead of IPF, may have significant therapeutic consequences, with the initiation of anti-inflammatory or immunosuppressive drugs instead of antifibrotic therapy or vice versa. They proposed future work should test the performance of these guidelines to differentiate HP from other ILDs in diverse and prospective cohorts, with an additional focus on developing robust studies that can answer the PICO questions stated in each guideline [1, 5, 16].

7 Future Directions

The ATS/JRS/ALAT 2020 guideline committee recognized an urgent need to improve knowledge on several topics, including (1) understanding the nature and pathophysiology of HP, (2) diagnostic approaches, (3) disease behavior and natural history, and (4) therapeutic approaches. Key questions on pathophysiology include genetic susceptibility and both host and environmental factors. For diagnostic approaches, important needs include the validation and standardization of questionnaires, BAL lymphocytosis threshold, specific antibodies, and biomarkers. In addition, new techniques like genomic classifiers and artificial intelligence to improve diagnosis and prognosis need to be assessed. Questions about disease behavior range from prevention to the phenotyping of HP. Regarding phenotyping, the differences between predominantly inflammatory and fibrotic subtypes are important questions. Finally, now that this guideline has established a standardized diagnostic approach to HP, future work needs to address the management of the different subtypes of HP in clinical trials and other researches [1].

References

1. Raghu G, Remy-Jardin M, Ryerson CJ, et al. Diagnosis of hypersensitivity pneumonitis in adults. An official ATS/JRS/ALAT clinical practice guideline. Am J Respir Crit Care Med. 202(3):e36–69.
2. Lacasse Y, Selman M, Costabel U, Dalphin JC, Ando M, Morell F, et al.; HP Study Group. Clinical diagnosis of hypersensitivity pneumonitis. Am J Respir Crit Care Med. 2003;168:952–958.
3. Walsh SLF, Wells AU, Desai SR, et al. Multicentre evaluation of multidisciplinary team meeting agreement on diagnosis in diffuse parenchymal lung disease: a case-cohort study. Lancet Respir Med. 2016;4(7):557–65.
4. Kaul B, Cottin V, Collard HR, et al. Variability in global prevalence of interstitial lung disease. Front Med (Lausanne). 2021;8:751181.
5. Fernández Pérez ER, Travis WD, Lynch DA, et al. Diagnosis and evaluation of hypersensitivity pneumonitis CHEST guideline and expert panel report. Chest. 2021;160(2):e97–e156.
6. Tomioka H, Miyazaki Y, Inoue Y, et al. Japanese clinical practice guide 2022 for hypersensitivity pneumonitis. Respir Investig. 2024;62(1):16–43.
7. Ryerson CJ, Corte TJ, Lee JS, Richeldi L, Walsh SLF, Myers JL, et al. A standardized diagnostic ontology for fibrotic interstitial lung disease: an international working group perspective. Am J Respir Crit Care Med. 2017;196:1249–54.
8. Okamoto T, Miyazaki Y, Ogura T, et al. Nationwide epidemiological survey of chronic hypersensitivity pneumonitis in Japan. Respir Investig. 2013;51(3):191–9.
9. Ohnishi H, Miyamoto S, Kawase S, et al. Seasonal variation of serum KL-6 concentrations is greater in patients with hypersensitivity pneumonitis. BMC Pulm Med. 2014;14:129.
10. Shirai T, Tanino Y, Nikaido T, et al. Screening and diagnosis of acute and chronic bird-related hypersensitivity pneumonitis by serum IgG and IgA antibodies to bird antigens with ImmunoCAP®. Allergol Int. 2021;70(2):208–14.
11. Raghu G, Remy-Jardin M, Richeldi L, et al. Idiopathic pulmonary fibrosis (an update) and progressive pulmonary fibrosis in adults: an official ATS/ERS/JRS/ALAT clinical practice guideline. Am J Respir Crit Care Med. 2022;205(9):e18–47.
12. Raghu G, Remy-Jardin M, Myers JL, et al. Diagnosis of idiopathic pulmonary fibrosis. An official ATS/ERS/JRS/ALAT clinical practice guideline. Am J Respir Crit Care Med. 2018;198(5):e44–68.
13. Marinescu DC, Raghu G, Remy-Jardin M, et al. Integration and application of clinical practice guidelines for the diagnosis of idiopathic pulmonary fibrosis and fibrotic hypersensitivity pneumonitis. Chest. 2022;162(3):614–29.
14. Marinescu DC, Hague CJ, Muller NL, et al. Integration and application of radiologic patterns from clinical practice guidelines on idiopathic pulmonary fibrosis and fibrotic hypersensitivity pneumonitis. Chest. 2023;164(6):1466–75.
15. Takei R, Yamano Y, Kataoka K, Yokoyama T, Matsuda T, Kimura T, Ozasa M, Fukuoka J, Johkoh T, Kondoh Y. New guideline diagnosis of fibrotic hypersensitivity pneumonitis in idiopathic pulmonary fibrosis. Am J Respir Crit Care Med. 2021;204(5):603–5.
16. Buendia-Roldan I, Aguilar-Duran H, Johannson KA, et al. Comparing the performance of two recommended criteria for establishing a diagnosis for hypersensitivity pneumonitis. Am J Respir Crit Care Med. 2021;204(7):865–8.

Chapter 5
Antigen Exposure Assessment

What Is Antigen Exposure Assecement in Diagnosis of HP?

Masaru Ejima

1 Introduction

Identification of the causative antigen is important not only to increase confidence in the diagnosis of hypersensitivity pneumonitis (HP), but also to improve the prognosis of HP by appropriate antigen avoidance. Antigens are identified by history taking, antigen questionnaires, immunological evaluation using antigen-specific antibodies and lymphocyte stimulation tests, antigen avoidance tests, provocation tests, and environmental surveys. However, standardization of these various evaluation methods is not easy, and antigen identification remains a major challenge in the management of diffuse lung disease. This chapter outlines the significance of antigen identification and exposure assessment, and proposes adaptations for the development of the antigen questionnaire, antigen identification confidence, and exposure assessment form in Japan.

2 Importance of Antigen Identification

The causative antigen has not been identified in 30–50% of cases [1]. This may depend on the type of HP in addition to the fact that evaluation methods for antigen identification have not yet been established. Nonfibrotic HP is often associated with cough, fever, increased inflammatory response, and worsening radiological findings as an acute reaction to antigen exposure. HP, especially those originating from the occupational environment, is often of an acute form due to high antigen levels. Together with temporal evaluation, such as symptoms appearing during work and

M. Ejima (✉)
Department of Respiratory Medicine, Musashino Red Cross Hospital, Tokyo, Japan

Y. Miyazaki (ed.), *Hypersensitivity Pneumonitis*, Respiratory Disease Series: Diagnostic Tools and Disease Managements,
https://doi.org/10.1007/978-981-96-7983-6_5

abating on weekends and long vacations, it is easy to find the cause in the environment. The symptoms of the disease diminish in the course of repeated acute symptoms (recurrent type), but it is easy to estimate the antigen according to acute clinical pictures. On the other hand, fibrotic HP progresses gradually without acute symptoms (insidious type), so it is not easy to estimate the causative antigen. Antigen identification is a particular clinical challenge in fibrotic HP, which can progress chronically and have a poor prognosis.

The first importance of antigen identification is to increase the pretest probability of HP diagnosis and to increase the diagnostic confidence. In both the 2020 ATS/JRS/ALAT and CHEST guidelines, antigen identification is included in the algorithm for determining confidence in HP diagnosis as a major criterion, along with other criteria such as imaging findings, lymphocyte fraction in **bronchoalveolar lavage** (BAL) fluid, and pathology findings [1, 2]. The guidelines aim to diagnose HP with a minimum of invasiveness. The 2020 ATS/JRS/ALAT guidelines have an algorithm that allows a diagnosis of HP with a high degree of confidence without evaluation of pathology, based on typical imaging findings and lymphocyte proliferation in BAL fluid, if the antigen is estimated during the history taking. The CHEST guidelines suggest that BAL for diagnostic purposes is unnecessary if the antigen is clearly identified and the imaging findings are typical. A multicenter prospective study examined the contribution of antigen identification to diagnosis [3–5]. In a cohort of 400 cases with respiratory illnesses, including 116 cases of HP, identification of the causative antigen was a particularly high odds ratio predictor of diagnosis among several clinical parameters, including precipitating antibodies, recurrent symptoms, and onset of symptoms after antigen exposure. In a retrospective study examining the risk of developing interstitial pneumonia in 6920 pigeon keepers, pigeon keeping was a higher risk factor compared to the control group. Furthermore, in a report of 46 cases of IPF diagnosed with HP, 43% of the cases were changed to HP, mainly due to close examination of antigen exposure. Therefore, exposure to antigens that are risk factors for the development of the disease should be thoroughly investigated for the diagnosis of HP. As part of the evaluation of new interstitial lung diseases (ILDs), it is recommended that all patients be interviewed for antigen exposure.

The second importance of antigen identification is its prognostic impact. There have been several reports of poor prognosis with unidentified antigens. In a single-center observational study of 142 patients with chronic HP, being antigen unspecified was an independent poor prognostic factor with an HR of 1.76 (95% CI 1.01–3.07) in a survival analysis adjusted for age, smoking history, respiratory function, and presence of fibrosis, and median survival was significantly worse in the antigen-unspecified group (4.88 vs. 8.75 years) [6]. In another retrospective cohort study of 202 patients with HP, a survival analysis adjusted for age, gender, and effort lung capacity showed a poor prognosis with a HR of 2.08 (95% CI 1.02–4.24). When antigen exposure was appropriately avoided, forced vital capacity improved significantly in nonfibrotic HP and showed a trend toward improvement even in fibrotic HP [7]. In another retrospective cohort of 72 cases of acute HP, 15% became chronic, and antigen unspecified was reported as an independent risk factor [8]. Furthermore, nonfibrotic HP with complete antigen avoidance by relocation was reported to be free from relapse and fibrosis [9]. Patients with fibrotic HP who were able to avoid antigens were reported to have a good prognosis [10]. Early antigen identification is important to improve prognosis through appropriate antigen avoidance.

3 Antigen Identification Procedure and Confidence Level

3.1 Antigen Identification Procedure

Surveys on antigen exposure should be conducted by consensus, with multiple endpoints being evaluated [11, 12]. It is desirable to conduct a multidisciplinary team approach that includes medical personnel and experts in the evaluation and improvement of the environment, based on the results of medical history and antigen questionnaire evaluation, improvement by antigen avoidance, environmental survey, immunological evaluation, and challenge tests. However, it is difficult in real-world clinical practice, because each of the evaluation items has issues in standardization and the training of experts. The CHEST guideline proposes five steps to continue the antigen exposure survey and to narrow down the candidates [2]. It consists of an exposure assessment, an evaluation of antigen type and source, a likelihood assessment of antigen identification, a team-based evaluation, and a site environmental assessment. In the case of unidentified antigens, improvement of clinical findings by antigen avoidance and environmental surveys at work and home are helpful. In view of the above, antigen identification in clinical practice is primary implemented by using the antigen questionnaire as a screening tool to pick up a wide range of causative antigens, and the suspected antigens are scrutinized by taking a medical history and other comprehensive evaluation, including antigen-specific antibody testing, provocation testing, antigen avoidance, and environmental studies.

3.2 Confidence Level of Antigen Identification

The degree of confidence in the causative antigen varies from case to case. For example, if a bird breeder shows typical imaging findings of HP and the findings improve with discontinuation of the breeding, there is a high degree of confidence in attributing antigen exposure to bird breeding. On the other hand, agricultural work is an environment of antigen exposure, but it is not a sufficient history, because there are many possible antigens such as microorganisms, fertilizers, birds, and plants. Similarly, it is difficult to be confident of a causative antigen for less convincing candidates obtained by interview, such as mold in the bathroom, use of down products, or birds flying into the living environment.

The 2020 ATS/JRS/ALAT guidelines do not specify the level of confidence [1]. The presence or absence of antigen exposure is evaluated as positive or negative and judged by a detailed interview, antigen-specific antibody test, and inhalation induction test, but the criteria for positive exposure are not clearly defined. It would be an overestimation to base the decision on the interview and antibody test alone. The clinical picture and reproduction of the disease should be shown to suggest an association between antigen and disease. For example, even if there is a known and obvious exposure, such as a bird breeder or mushroom grower, it is not considered positive unless the patient can show worsening of clinical findings consistent with the time of exposure.

The CHEST guideline uses an algorithm with a more detailed flow that divides the contribution of antigen exposure to the diagnosis of HP into three categories: identified, indeterminate, and unidentified [2]. Identified refers to a situation in which there is sufficient evidence of an association between the causative antigen and the disease, that is, sufficient evidence of worsening of clinical findings due to antigen exposure, reproduction of the disease, or improvement due to avoidance. Indeterminate refers to a case in which the antigen is suspected as the causative antigen, but the association with symptoms cannot be demonstrated and is inconclusive. This applies to situations in which there is a suspected antigen by interview or antibody test, but the clinical findings coinciding with the time of exposure, improvement by avoidance of the suspected antigen, or reproduction by induction tests, etc., have not been obtained. Unidentified refers to cases in which the causative antigen cannot be estimated by detailed antigen exposure interviews and clinical evaluation, and requires continuous interviewing. Continuous interview and examination should be conducted to identify causative antigens.

We present a draft evaluation criterion for judging the degree of antigen confidence using the Antigen Exposure Assessment Form (Table 5.1). For each candidate antigen based on the antigen questionnaire (A) and antibody test (B), the association between antigen and disease is demonstrated by showing worsening (C1) or improvement with intervention (C2) consistent with the time of exposure, or by replication by provocation testing (D). These items are proposed for the definition of positive and negative in the 2020 ATS/JRS/ALAT guidelines and identified, indeterminate, and unidentified in the CHEST guidelines. For example, if symptoms, serum markers, lung capacity, and imaging worsen (C1) or improve with avoidance from the environment (C2) coinciding with the time of use of the humidifier (A), the patient is judged as exposure positive and indeterminate. If house mold is suspected as an antigen by interview and antibody test (A) (B), and if there is worsening of findings during the summer (C1), and if there is no relapse or progression of the disease by avoiding the home or removing the mold by house cleaning (C2), the case is considered exposure positive and identified. The proposed criteria are designed to deal with the insidious type that is difficult to identify antigens. Prospective validation should be conducted to develop criteria that will enable standardized evaluation at many facilities, not just at specialized centers.

Table 5.1 Antigen exposure assessment form

Antigen exposure assessment form Date of evaluation:					
Screening of antigen exposure					
		Grading of clinical significance (G1 ~ G4)			
Antigen	A. Questionnaire and history taking[a]	B. Immunological findings	C. Association with clinical picture	D. Reproducibility	Grade
Fungi/molds	☐ Location ( ) ☐ Moldy odor ☐ Rooms with poor sunlight ☐ Rooms with dampness ☐ Leaks and flooding ☐ Wooden structure 20 years or more ☐ Others ( )	☐ Anti-*T.asahii*-Ab positive ☐ Others ( )	C1 Suggests deterioration due to increased antigen exposure [b] ☐ Worsening with contact ☐ Seasonal aggravation ☐ Worsening by return to environment C2 Suggests improvement due to decreased antigen exposure ☐ Antigen avoidance test positive[b] ☐ Stabilization after antigen removal[c]	Individual provocation test[d] ☐ positive	☐ G1 ☐ G2 ☐ G3 ☐ G4
Avian	**Contact with birds** ☐ History of breeding ☐ Neighborhood breeding, sheds, nests ☐ Habits of feeding and contact ☐ Flying, feathers, droppings in the yard **Feather products** **(Down jacket or feather duvet, etc)** ☐ Use by patient ☐ Use only by family members ☐ Storing **Poultry manure fertilizer** ☐ Use at home ☐ Use in neighborhood ☐ **Others** ( )	Bird-specific IgG ☐ Pigeon positive ☐ Budgerigar positive ☐ Others ( )	C1 Suggests deterioration due to increased antigen exposure [b] ☐ Worsening with contact ☐ Seasonal aggravation ☐ Worsening by return to environment C2 Suggests improvement due to decreased antigen exposure ☐ Antigen avoidance test positive[b] ☐ Stabilization after antigen removal[c]	Individual provocation test[d] ☐ Positive	☐ G1 ☐ G2 ☐ G3 ☐ G4

(continued)

Table 5.1 (continued)

Antigen exposure assessment form Date of evaluation:					
Humidifier	☐ Ultrasonic type ☐ Heating type ☐ Other types ( )		C1 Suggests deterioration due to increased antigen exposure [b] ☐ Worsening with contact ☐ Seasonal aggravation ☐ Worsening by return to environment C2 Suggests improvement due to decreased antigen exposure ☐ Antigen avoidance test positive[b] ☐ Stabilization after antigen removal[c]	Individual provocation test[d] ☐ Positive	☐ G1 ☐ G2 ☐ G3 ☐ G4
Others ( )	Details ( )	Details ( )	C1 Suggests deterioration due to increased antigen exposure [b] ☐ Worsening with contact ☐ Seasonal aggravation ☐ Worsening by return to environment C2 Suggests improvement due to decreased antigen exposure ☐ Antigen avoidance test positive[b] ☐ Stabilization after antigen removal[c]	Individual provocation test[d] ☐ Positive	☐ G1 ☐ G2 ☐ G3 ☐ G4

Antigen Identification Methods Using Antigen Exposure Assessment Forms:
First, to narrow down the target antigens, A is evaluated by antigen questionnaire and detailed history taking, and B is evaluated by immunological findings including antigen-specific IgG tests. For each antigen candidate, C (presence of a clinical picture indicating an association between antigen and disease) and D (reproducibility by antigen exposure) are evaluated. The grading of clinical significance for each antigen is determined as follows:

Grading of Clinical Significance

G1 (not evident): B, C, D all negative: (CHEST: **unidentified**, ATS/JRS/ALAT: **negative**)

G2 (weak suspicion): B or C1 or C2 positive: (CHEST: **indeterminate**, ATS/JRS/ALAT: **negative**)

G3 (strong suspicion); B + C1, B + C2, C1 + C2: (CHEST: **indeterminate**, ATS/JRS/ALAT: **positive**)

G4 (confirmed); B + C1 + C2, D: (CHEST**: identified**, ATS/JRS/ALAT: **positive**)

[a]Evaluate by antigen questionnaire and detailed medical history interview

[b]Confirm improvement with antigen avoidance for 2–4 weeks in multiple findings including symptoms, blood findings (AaDO2, KL-6, SP-D, WBC, CRP, LDH, etc.), lung function, and radiological findings. Criteria for antigen avoidance testing in hospitalization [43]: Positive results in at least 2 of the following criteria are used as references: VC 3% or greater increase, WBC 3% or greater decrease, KL-6 13% or greater decrease, and both inpatient and outpatient are acceptable for evaluation

[c]This evaluation is based on a negative antigen avoidance test or not performed. Short antigen avoidance tests do not have high diagnostic sensitivity especially for insidious type. After removal of the suspicious antigen, the patient should be followed up until the same season of the next year to ensure that there is no progression of symptoms, lung function, or imaging findings. Reference findings for judgment are a decrease in %FVC of less than 3% and the absence of progressive fibrosis or the appearance of ground-glass shadows on HRCT

[d]Refers to a selective environmental challenge test or inhalation provocation test with the suspected antigen

[e]For the relevant antigen, the deterioration of one of the following items during the exposure period is judged: symptoms (fever, cough, shortness of breath), serum markers (KL-6, SP-D, LDH, CRP, etc.), lung function, and radiological findings

4 Interview for Antigen Identification

4.1 Epidemiological Data Required for the Medical Interview

The organization of causative antigens is essential to the interview for antigen identification. The type and amount of antigens present in the living environment, the duration of exposure, and the sensitivity of the individual to the antigen are all involved in the development of HP. Epidemiological data in Japan are important, because the types and frequency of HP vary widely from country to country and region to region.

As an epidemiological study corresponding to acute HP, 835 cases were accumulated from 1980 to 1989, of which 74.4% were summer type, 8.1% farmer's lung, 4.3% ventilator pneumonia, and 4.1% bird-feeder disease [13]. A national survey of 222 cases of chronic HP from 2000 to 2009 included 60.4% with bird related, 14.9% with summer type, 11.3% with home related, 1.8% with farmer's lung, 1.4% with painter's lung, and 10.4% with others [14]. The incidence of occupational HP has been reported overseas to be changing with changes in industrial and living environments [15]. Epidemiological studies of occupational HP in the UK from 1996 to 2015 showed a decreasing trend in farmer's lung and mushroom grower's lung, while the frequency of mechanic's lung was increasing.

In view of the above, it is essential to conduct thorough interviews and evaluations of frequently causative antigens, such as bird related, summer type, and housing related. Evaluation of antigens in response to changes in industry and living environments is also important. There is a need to accumulate case reports on the causative environment and antigens of HP in Japan, and to build a resource of lists of causative antigens available to clinicians [16].

4.2 Classification of Causative Antigens Based on Environmental Source

When interviewing exposure antigens, the specific pathogenic environment in which the causative antigen is present should be asked. In other words, it is necessary to organize the causative antigens by environmental source. However, classification of the causative antigen is often made according to the type of antigen (i.e., microorganism, protein of animal or plant origin, or chemical substance) or diagnostic name (i.e., bird related, residence related, occupational) [17, 18]. This classification method is not practical from the viewpoint of medical interview. Table 5.2 organizes the antigens by causative environment, and supplementary information lists the corresponding disease names. Environmental sources can be roughly classified into four categories: water contamination (ventilation, residential, occupational), plant related (farming and food processing, cereals, wood), animal related (birds, other animals, food processing), and industrial inorganic (chemicals, metals, drugs). Supplementary information for each category is provided below.

Table 5.2 Classification of causative antigens based on environmental source

Environmental sources	Specific environment	Name of specific disease
Water contamination Ventilation	Source of microbial bioaerosol: Contaminated water in humidifiers and air conditioners, portable air conditioner, fan cooler, dehumidifier	Humidifier lung, air-conditioning disease, ventilation pneumonitis
Residential	House leaks and flooding, dirt and corrosion in bathrooms and kitchens, contamination of wooden furniture, tatami mats, carpets, sofas, and others upholstered furniture, wind instrument	Summer-type HP, home-related HP, wind-instrument alveolitis, bagpipe lung
	Moisture and mold in hot tubs (recirculating tubs, jetted tubs), Contamination in saunas	Hot tub lung, sauna taker's lung
Occupational	Contamination of metalworking fluids (cooling water and lubricating fluids) in automotive plants, sewage treatment, plumbing operations	Machine operator's lung, sewer worker's lung
Plant related Agricultural work and food processing	Moldy hay, grains, stored grass, sugar cane, sugar mills, confectionery manufacturing, tobacco, mushroom spores, compost for mushroom cultivation, greenhouse cultivation of orchids, roses, cucumbers, etc., compost, mold on potatoes, bell peppers, grapes, other vegetables and fruits, breweries, coffee bean dust, tea cultivation, green tea powder.	Farmer's lung, bagassosis, tobacco grower's lung, mushroom grower's lung, greenhouse worker's lung, compost lung, potato riddler's lung, paprika slicer's lung, wine grower's lung, coffee worker's lung, tea grower's lung
Grains	Grain flour (wheat, malt, beans, etc.), Flour mite contamination of flour, dried bonito flakes, cheese, etc., Weevil-infested flour, moldy barley, bakery and bread-making yeast, confectionery product	Flour-dust alveolitis, Miller's lung, wheat-weevil lung, malt worker's lung, baker's lung
Wood	Timber harvesting, maple bark peeling, wood chips and dust from woodworking including hobby (diy), woodworkers, sequoia sawdust, wood pulp, wood drying and rotting, fallen leaves, dead leaves, thatch roofs, cork mold	Wood trimmer's disease, maple bark disease, woodworker's lung, wood fiber alveolitis, sequoiosis, wood pulp worker's disease, dry rot lung, thatched-roof lung, cork worker's lung
Others	Contamination of plaster exterior walls, cosmetic powder (argan cake), raw garbage	Stucco worker's lung, argan cake HP, waste sorter's lung
Animal related Avian	Raising birds, Use of down products (down duvets, pillows, down jackets), Contact with bird droppings and feathers, Use of poultry manure fertilizers	Bird fancier's lung, feather-duvet lung, bird-related HP

(continued)

Table 5.2 (continued)

Environmental sources	Specific environment	Name of specific disease
Others animals	Animal fur, Hair, and excrement of laboratory animals (rats and other rodents), excrement of bats, cocoon scraping and scurf removal in sericulture, foot care	Furrier's lung, laboratory worker's HP, sausage worker's lung, bat lung, silkworm rearer's lung, footcare alveolitis
Food processing	Cheese mold, sausage making, fish meat and fish meal dust, oyster shell powder, milk powder, milk (infant)	Cheese washer's lung, salami producer's lung, fish food lung, fish meal worker's lung, oyster-shell HP, Heiner syndrome
Inorganic materials Chemicals	Isocyanates (polyurethane foam, rubber spray, lacquer paint, automobile maintenance, castings), acid anhydride curing agents such as epoxy resins in plastic processing, acrylic resins for dental materials, Bordeaux solution (agricultural chemicals including copper sulfate for grapes), coolants for laser hair removal, polyester powder	Painter's lung, isocyanate alveolitis, acid anhydride alveolitis, methacrylate alveolitis, vineyard sprayer's lung, hair-remover lung
Metals	Zinc fume, cobalt, zirconium, trimethylindium, beryllium	Giant cell pneumonitis, zinc-fumes alveolitis, beryllium HP
Drugs	Penicillins, cephems, methotrexate, interferon alpha, pravastatin, etc.,	Drug-induced HP

First, water contamination is a source of microbial bioaerosol, which is increasingly being caused by ventilation equipment, especially humidifiers. Cooling air conditioners with water tanks, cooling fans, and dehumidifiers are similar sources. Regarding the living environment as a source of water contamination, it is important to ask the development of summer type and home related. The main cause, *Trichosporon asahii*, is found in wooden houses built more than 20 years ago [19]. *Trichosporon ashii* breeds on rotten wood, carpets, tatami mats, bedding, kitchens, washrooms, and bathrooms where sunlight and ventilation are poor and humidity are high, which is an important part of the interview. In recent years, the environment where *Trichosporon* can easily breed has been increasing regardless of the season or region due to the improvement of heating systems and airtightness of buildings [20]. Questions regarding the contamination of wind instruments [21] and hot-tub lungs caused by *Mycobacterium avium* in circulatory bathtubs and jet baths [22] are also asked.

Among plant-related origins, farmer's lung in dairy and livestock industries that handle stored grass [23], mushroom grower's lung caused by spores and microorganisms that proliferate in the growing environment [24], and greenhouse grower's lung caused in hot and humid greenhouses [25] have been reported. The disease may occur in fruit selection in poorly ventilated warehouses [26], sorting of vegetables and fruits, coffee bean dust, and tea factory and tea powder, with plant-derived proteins and attached microorganisms as the causative antigens. In cereals, the disease may be caused by wheat itself, mold, mites, and weevils attached to the grain, or by yeast from baking [27]. In wood, woodworker's lung is caused by inhalation of microorganisms on wet wood chips from timber harvesting and carpentry and woodworking craftsmen's work [28]. In recent years, there have been cases due to inhalation of wood chips from hobbyist woodworking (DIY).

For animal-related cases, a detailed interview for the most frequent avian-associated antigens should be conducted. Interviews include direct exposure due to bird keeping, presence of bird nests and aviaries, bird keeping in the neighborhood, bird feeding, and presence of bird flyovers, feather and bird droppings in the home's yard. The use of feather products and poultry manure fertilizers should also be checked. Acute cases of feather duvet lung are occasionally experienced [29]. It is useful to ask about bird flights to the home' yard to suspect exposure to avian antigens [30]. The group of patients who had high levels of bird antigen in their homes reported significantly more responses to questionnaires about birds flying to their balconies and yards and about seeing feathers and bird droppings. A research study at the same institution found that bird antigens were present in the air and in indoor dust in houses tens of meters away from birdhouses, in houses next to small bird stores, and in residential settings where there were many wild birds [31]. In food processing, there have been cases caused by mold in cheese, sausage, and fish meat, and it is desirable to hear extensively about food processing as well.

As for inorganic materials in industry, there are many reports of isocyanate-associated outbreaks. Isocyanates are commercially available as foaming and spraying agents for polyurethane foams and are used for thermal insulation. It is also used as a hardener in automotive coatings, furniture and floor coatings, and anticorrosion coatings, and is commercially available as a spray agent. It is important to ask about isocyanate products at home as well as at work [32]. Epoxy resins are also used as rust inhibitors and are commercially available as paints and spray agents, and can be a causative antigen. There is also onset due to inhalation of metal fumes from welders and dust inhalation from metal grinding [33, 34]. The occupational environment should be thoroughly inquired. It is also helpful to have the patient bring a material/chemical use list or data sheet, especially if occupational exposure to inorganic materials is suspected.

4.3 History Taking and Antigen Questionnaire

Comprehensive and standardized history taking is desirable but practically difficult, because of the differences in experience among clinicians and the time constraints of daily clinical practice. Suspected exposures should be assessed for duration, intensity, frequency, and involvement in symptoms, as well as for changes in exposure due to seasonal changes or temporary activities (e.g., farming, changing clothes, moving to a summer or vacation home, hobbies.). Continuous interviews may reveal new exposures. When taking a medical history, open-ended questions,

Table 5.3 Antigen questionnaire

This is an environmental questionnaire for possible causes of lung disease. Date of evaluation: ( )
Residential environment
(1) Home address: (___)
(2) Age of building: (___), Years of residence: (___), Floor: (___), Construction (Wooden, others)
(3) Rooms with poor lighting: (No, Yes; which room? ___)
(4) Rooms with dampness: (No, Yes; which room? ___)
(5) Musty smells: (No, Yes)
(6) Visible or significant mold or mildew: (No, Yes; where? baths, washers, washbasins, kitchen, windows, walls, wooden furniture, tatami mats, qquilt and mattress, carpets, others: ___)
(7) Are there any facilities? (circulating bathtub, jacuzzi, mist sauna, custom of storing bath water, none)
(8) Is there a history of water damage, moisture, leaks, or flooding? (No, Yes)
(9) Are there any of the following near your home? (fields, rivers, wetlands, none)
Lifestyle
(1) Use of humidifiers: (No, Yes; which types? ultrasonic, vaporized, hybrid, heated, integrated air purifier)
When or which season to start using it? ___)
Are they cleaned regularly? (No, Yes: how often? ___)
(2) Use of air conditioners: (No, Yes; how many years since purchase? ___)
When or which season to start using it? ___)
Are they cleaned regularly? (No, Yes: how often? ___)
(3) Use of feather duvet: (current, former, never)
The period of time that you used duvet? (from ___ to ___)
Do any of your family members currently use duvet? (No, Yes)
(4) Use of down or feather products: (jackets, pillows, dusters, stuffed bird, others: ___ , none)
(5) Use of poultry manure fertilizer: (no, use at home, use in neiborhood, unknown)
(6) History of breeding birds: (never, former, current)
When, what kind of birds, and how many birds were kept? (___)
(7) Do you have a neighbor raising birds, or are there aviaries or bird nests nearby? (No, Yes, unknown)
(8) Are there any birds flying, feathers, or bird droppings in the yard or on the balcony? (No, Yes)
(9) Do you have contact with birds or feed birds? (No, Yes)
(10) Do you currently keep any animals other than birds? (No, Yes: animal species: ___)

(continued)

Occupational history

Age (from ________ to ________): Job title (________________) Job description (________________)
Age (from ________ to ________): Job title (________________) Job description (________________)
Age (from ________ to ________): Job title (________________) Job description (________________)

Place a tick in the boxes below if you have been exposed to these on a regular basis.

☐ Agricultural work, growing vegetables, fruits, flowers, and mushrooms
☐ Hay, livestock feed, compost
☐ Pruning and planting of garden trees
☐ Grain flour for bread, confectionery, noodle, etc.,
☐ Vegetable sorting
☐ Tea or coffee bean powder
☐ Cleaning up fallen leaves and debris
☐ Moldy cork, lumber, bark
☐ Wood chips, wood dust, DIY
☐ Wind instruments
☐ Cooling Fan with Water Tank, dehumidifiers
☐ Food processing for sausage and cheese production, etc.,
☐ Animal hair and excrement
☐ Coolant and lubricant in machining
☐ Metal dust from welding and grinding
☐ Painting or spraying with isocyanate, such as polyurethane foam or lacquer

Do you have any other jobs or hobbies that may inhale mold or dust?

(____)

What do you think triggers the symptoms (cough, breathlessness, fever) in the above?

(____)

illustrations to aid the patient's recall, and interviews with family members and caregivers can help to increase the information. It is also helpful to ask patients to take pictures of their workplace or living environment, or even to check their surroundings by conducting a geographic search on the web [2].

In contrast, the antigen questionnaire may provide a means of overcoming the problems of reliability, reproducibility, and time constraints of medical history taking. In a systematic review of the usefulness of antigen questionnaires (although only two reports of a small number of cases were included), the questionnaire seems useful as the combined antibody test and inhalation provocation test (59% vs. 65%, RR 0.90, 95% CI 0.65–1.24). The more items on the antigen questionnaire, the more useful it was in identifying antigens [35]. In view of the above, it is recommended that the antigen questionnaire be used first as a tool for a comprehensive interview to identify a wide range of possible causative antigens, and then the obtained suspected antigens be examined closely by taking a medical history to determine if they are the target of further examination as causative antigens.

The content of the antigen questionnaire should include three elements: a list of causative antigens based on regional characteristics, an occupational exposure questionnaire, and a living environment questionnaire [2]. Although international standardization is difficult, it is necessary to develop an antigen questionnaire in Japan based on epidemiology and case reports. Although there are several reports of antigen questionnaires in foreign countries, the validity of the questionnaires has not been verified [17, 18, 36]. A report using the Delphi method summarized the important questions to ask when suspecting chronic HP [36]. The questions were distilled into 16 key questions that included moisture and mold odors as microbial sources, animal- and plant-derived proteins including feather products and wood dust, and inorganic materials such as isocyanates, vapors, gases, and fumes. The questionnaire also asks about the duration of exposure to the suspected antigen and the timing of the onset of symptoms. With regard to fungi, some reports have indicated a questionnaire to determine fungal outbreaks in the home and indications for home environmental surveys [37, 38]. The report proposes screening questions for fungal outbreaks that includes moisture and water damage in the house, mold odor and development, the presence of condensation, poorly ventilated rooms, and ventilation systems.

The proposed antigen questionnaire in Japan is shown in Table 5.3. The questionnaire was designed as a comprehensive antigen questionnaire, including the frequently asked questions on bird-related questions, summer, home-related questions, and ventilators, as well as a checklist of sources reported in Japan, which are summarized in Table 5.2, and open-ended questions. All patients with ILD are asked about the environment of antigen exposure at the time of initial examination in order to actively suspect the possibility of HP.

5 Environmental Survey

The environmental survey, by actually visiting the home or workplace, complements environmental exposures that cannot be obtained from a medical interview alone. Environmental surveys may be useful in identifying causative antigens, sampling microorganisms from the environment, and even suggesting measures to improve the environment, but the evidence is limited. In clinical practice, it may be indicated in cases of unspecified antigens or repeated exacerbations of the disease.

There are limited reports that present methodologies on the practical assessment of environments and improvement measures. When suspecting fungal infections in the residence, how an environmental survey specialist conducts a field survey has been reported [37]. A building survey (walkthrough) evaluates the condition of moisture, ventilation, drainage, and ventilation systems. Visual observation includes evaluation of indoor and outdoor walls, condensation, water and furniture, bedding, carpeting, air conditioning units, fungal hotbeds including basements and attics, and yard conditions. Microorganisms are sampled at suspected locations. A case report proposed a detailed environmental survey in chronic HP with repeated relapses [39]. In the report, among multiple candidates in the home suspected by the interview, environmental survey revealed that corroded wood in the home was strongly suspected as the cause, leading to a diagnosis of home-related HP. Examples of environmental surveys related to bird antigens include the discovery of a bird nest in the outdoor hood of a ventilation fan, a sofa and fluffer made of down, bird droppings inhaled while cleaning the roof in the apartment management. As a point of reference, residential environment surveys and intervention approaches have been reported for bronchial asthma and would be useful for HP [40, 41].

Regarding environmental sampling, there is a small study of 19 cases in which samples collected by swabbing were used to identify microorganisms by PCR and antigen identification by the octarony method with patient sera [42]. The importance of field investigations is discussed, as specimens obtained from environmental sampling have a higher concordance rate between causative microorganisms and patient sera than those obtained from panel testing of sera. It is also important to actively evaluate the environment and attempt to identify antigens in the early stages of the disease, when antigen exposure can cause symptoms.

There are no qualified experts in the field of residential environment surveys in Japan, and staff training is also an issue. In addition, there are several private companies that evaluate fungi in the environment and undertake cleaning and removal work, and it is an issue to be considered how to collaborate and utilize these companies in the future.

6 Conclusion and Future Issues

This chapter outlines the significance of antigen identification in HP, a proposed evaluation of the confidence level of antigen identification, an organization of causative antigens for efficient interviewing of the antigen-exposed environment, a specific proposal for an antigen questionnaire, and the adaptation of environmental surveys. The following is a list of issues related to these issues that need to be resolved in the future.

- Standardization and validation of the antigen questionnaire in Japan.
- Validation of the antigen exposure assessment form.
- Establishment of a methodology for antigen identification in HP and its impact on prognosis.
- Investigation of the type, intensity, and duration of antigen exposure and its involvement in the development of HP.
- Establishment of information resource on antigens causing HP in Japan.
- Build evidence and train staff on the significance and methodology of environmental research.

References

1. Raghu G, Remy-Jardin M, Ryerson CJ, et al. Diagnosis of hypersensitivity pneumonitis in adults. An official ATS/JRS/ALAT clinical practice guideline. Am J Respir Crit Care Med. 2020;202:e36–69.
2. Fernández Pérez ER, Travis WD, Lynch DA, et al. Executive summary diagnosis and evaluation of hypersensitivity pneumonitis: CHEST guideline and expert panel report. Chest. 2021;S0012-3692(21):00686–3. https://doi.org/10.1016/j.chest.2021.03.066.
3. Lacasse Y, Selman M, Costabel U, et al. Clinical diagnosis of hypersensitivity pneumonitis. Am J Respir Crit Care Med. 2003;168:952–8.
4. Cramer C, Schlünssen V, Bendstrup E, et al. Risk of hypersensitivity pneumonitis and interstitial lung diseases among pigeon breeders. Eur Respir J. 2016;48:818–25.
5. Morell F, Villar A, Montero MÁ, et al. Chronic hypersensitivity pneumonitis in patients diagnosed with idiopathic pulmonary fibrosis: a prospective case-cohort study. Lancet Respir Med. 2013;1:685–94.
6. Fernández Pérez ER, Swigris JJ, Forssén AV, et al. Identifying an inciting antigen is associated with improved survival in patients with chronic hypersensitivity pneumonitis. Chest. 2013;144:1644–51.
7. De Sadeleer LJ, Hermans F, De Dycker E, et al. Effects of corticosteroid treatment and antigen avoidance in a large hypersensitivity pneumonitis cohort: a single-centre cohort study. J Clin Med. 2018;8:14.
8. Wang LJ, Cai HR, Xiao YL, et al. Clinical characteristics and outcomes of hypersensitivity pneumonitis: a population-based study in China. Chin Med J. 2019;132:1283–92.
9. Nishida T, Kawate E, Ishiguro T, Kanauchi T, Shimizu Y, Takayanagi N. Antigen avoidance and outcome of nonfibrotic and fibrotic hypersensitivity pneumonitis. ERJ Open Res. 2021;8:00474–2021.
10. Petnak T, Thongprayoon C, Baqir M, Ryu JH, Moua T. Antigen identification and avoidance on outcomes in fibrotic hypersensitivity pneumonitis. Eur Respir J. 2022;60:2101336.

11. Johannson KA, Barnes H, Bellanger AP, et al. Exposure assessment tools for hypersensitivity pneumonitis. An official American Thoracic Society Workshop Report. Ann Am Thorac Soc. 2020;17:1501–9.
12. Copeland CR, Collins BF, Salisbury ML. Identification and remediation of environmental exposures in patients with interstitial lung disease: evidence review and practical considerations. Chest. 2021;160:219–30.
13. Yoshida K, Suga M, Nishiura Y, et al. Occupational hypersensitivity pneumonitis in Japan: data on a nationwide epidemiological study. Occup Environ Med. 1995;52:570–4.
14. Okamoto T, Miyazaki Y, Ogura T, et al. Nationwide epidemiological survey of chronic hypersensitivity pneumonitis in Japan. Respir Investig. 2013;51:191–9.
15. Barber CM, Wiggans RE, Carder M, Agius R. Epidemiology of occupational hypersensitivity pneumonitis; reports from the SWORD scheme in the UK from 1996 to 2015. Occup Environ Med. 2017;74:528–30.
16. Lu J, Barnes H, Johannson KA. hpLung.com. [accessed 2021 Aug 10]. Available from: http://www.hplung.com/.
17. Vasakova M, Morell F, Walsh S, et al. Hypersensitivity pneumonitis: perspectives in diagnosis and management. Am J Respir Crit Care Med. 2017;196:680–9.
18. Petnak T, Moua T. Exposure assessment in hypersensitivity pneumonitis: a comprehensive review and proposed screening questionnaire. ERJ Open Res. 2020;6:00230–2020. https://doi.org/10.1183/23120541.00230-2020.
19. Ando M, Arima K, Yoneda R, et al. Japanese summer-type hypersensitivity pneumonitis. Geographic distribution, home environment, and clinical characteristics of 621 cases. Am Rev Respir Dis. 1991;144:765–9.
20. Ishikawa T, Kawasaki T, Shimaya K, et al. Familial summer-type hypersensitivity pneumonitis in summer and winter at the work place. Arerugi. 2017;66:1236–9. [In Japanese]
21. Møller J, Hyldgaard C, Kronborg-White SB, et al. Hypersensitivity pneumonitis among wind musicians – an overlooked disease? Eur Clin Respir J. 2017;4:1351268.
22. Tsuchiya N, Takayanagi N, Yoneda K, et al. Case of hot tub lung with confirmation of exacerbation following jet bath use. Nihon Kokyuki Gakkai Zasshi. 2008;46:726–31. [In Japanese]
23. Ishiguroa T, Takayanagia N, Yoneda K, et al. Farmer's lung diagnosed by inhalation provocation test performed in hospital room. Nihon Kokyuki Gakkai Zasshi. 2012;1:67–71. [In Japanese]
24. Rikimaru M, Tanino Y, Fukuhara A, et al. Two cases of hypersensitivity pneumonitis in mushroom workers. Japan J Sarcoidosis Vasc Diffuse Lung Dis. 2018;38:85–8. [In Japanese]
25. Amano Y, Enomoto M, Bando M, et al. Hypersensitity pneumonitis in a greenhouse rose grower. Nihon Kokyuki Gakkai Zasshi. 2009;47:960–4. [In Japanese]
26. Yasui H, Matsui T, Yokomura K, et al. Three cases of hypersensitivity pneumonitis in citrus farmers. Nihon Kokyuki Gakkai Zasshi. 2010;48:172–7. [In Japanese]
27. Shioya M, Otsuka M, Nishikiori H, et al. A case of hypersensitivity pneumonitis induced by homemade baker's yeast (Saccharomyces cerevisiae). Nihon Kokyuki Gakkai Zasshi. 2015;4:380–4. [In Japanese]
28. Mackiewicz B, Dutkiewicz J, Siwiec J, et al. Acute hypersensitivity pneumonitis in woodworkers caused by inhalation of birch dust contaminated with Pantoea agglomerans and Microbacterium barkeri. Ann Agric Environ Med. 2019;26:644–55.
29. Kondo K, Inase N, Ohtani Y, et al. A case of acute bird fancier's lung caused by feather duvet. Nihon Kokyuki Gakkai Zasshi. 2003;41:569–72. [In Japanese]
30. Sema M, Miyazaki Y, Tsutsui T, et al. Environmental levels of avian antigen are relevant to the progression of chronic hypersensitivity pneumonitis during antigen avoidance. Immun Inflamm Dis. 2018;6:154–62.
31. Kuramochi J, Inase N, Takayama K, Miyazaki Y, Yoshizawa Y. Detection of indoor and outdoor avian antigen in management of bird-related hypersensitivity pneumonitis. Allergol Int. 2010;59(2):223–8.

32. Tabata H, Mochizuki Y, Nakahara Y, et al. Hypersensitivity pneumonitis caused by isocyanate exposure during recreational painting. Nihon Kokyuki Gakkai Zasshi. 2009;47:1002–7. [In Japanese]
33. Miyazaki H, Hirata T, Shimane S, et al. A case of hypersensitivity pneumonitis caused by zinc fume. Nihon Kokyuki Gakkai Zasshi. 2006;44:985–9. [In Japanese]
34. Sakamoto O, Kosai S, Kohrogi H. A case of hard metal lung disease presenting a type of chronic hypersensitivity pneumonitis. Nihon Kokyuki Gakkai Zasshi. 2008;46:535–41. [In Japanese]
35. Jenkins AR, Chua A, Chami H, et al. Questionnaires or serum immunoglobulin G testing in the diagnosis of hypersensitivity pneumonitis among patients with interstitial lung disease. Ann Am Thorac Soc. 2021;18:130–47.
36. Barnes H, Morisset J, Molyneaux P, et al. A systematically derived exposure assessment instrument for chronic hypersensitivity pneumonitis. Chest. 2020;157:1506–12.
37. Chew GL, Horner WE, Kennedy K, et al. Environmental Allergens Workgroup. Procedures to assist health care providers to determine when home assessments for potential mold exposure are warranted. J Allergy Clin Immunol Pract. 2016;4:417–22.e2.
38. Storey E, Dangman KH, Schenck P, et al. Guidance for clinicians on the recognition and management of health effects related to mold exposure and moisture indoors. Farmington, CT: University of Connecticut Health Center, Division of Occupational and Environmental Medicine, Center for Indoor Environments and Health; 2004. Available from: https://www.epa.gov/mold/guidance-clinicians-recognition-and-management-health-effects-related-mold-exposure-and
39. Takayama K, Kuramochi J, Inase N. A case of summer-type hypersensitivity pneumonitis diagnosed after environmental investigation and a provocation test. Nihon Kokyuki Gakkai Zasshi. 2012;1:119–23. [In Japanese]
40. Morgan WJ, Crain EF, Gruchalla RS, et al. Inner-City Asthma Study Group. Results of a home-based environmental intervention among urban children with asthma. N Engl J Med. 2004;351:1068–80.
41. Delclos GL, Arif AA, Aday L, et al. Validation of an asthma questionnaire for use in healthcare workers. Occup Environ Med. 2006;63:173–9.
42. Millerick-May ML, Mulks MH, Gerlach J, et al. Hypersensitivity pneumonitis and antigen identification – an alternate approach. Respir Med. 2016;112:97–105.
43. Tsutsui T, Miyazaki Y, Okamoto T, et al. Antigen avoidance tests for diagnosis of chronic hypersensitivity pneumonitis. Respir Investig. 2015;53:217–24.

Chapter 6
Immunological Tests (Antigen-Specific IgG, Lymphocyte Proliferation Test)

What Is Immunologic Tests in Diagnosis of HP?

Tsuyoshi Shirai

1 Introduction

Hypersensitivity pneumonitis (HP) is an extrinsic allergic alveolitis caused by repeated inhalation of inciting antigen. The immunopathology of HP is not uniform, and it differs by subtype of the disease. Traditionally, HP has been classified into acute and chronic HP, though recent guidelines propose a new classification based on absence/presence of lung fibrosis, namely, nonfibrotic and fibrotic, the most important factor related to patients' prognosis.

Antigen-specific IgGs against the inciting antigen can be detected in the patients' serum and bronchoalveolar lavage fluid, which forms the immune complex, a key molecule in the pathophysiology of acute HP (nonfibrotic). Additionally, T-lymphocytes also play an important role in the disease; cell proliferation is observed when peripheral lymphocytes are stimulated with the inciting antigen.

The diagnosis of fibrotic HP (insidious type of chronic HP) can be quitechallenging, because it is often difficult to distinguish from other fibrotic interstitial lung diseases. Therefore, evaluation of the presence of these disease-specific immune responses is essential for the diagnosis of HP.

T. Shirai (✉)
Department of Respiratory Medicine, Institution of Science Tokyo, Tokyo, Japan
e-mail: tshipulm@tmd.ac.jp

Y. Miyazaki (ed.), *Hypersensitivity Pneumonitis*, Respiratory Disease Series: Diagnostic Tools and Disease Managements,
https://doi.org/10.1007/978-981-96-7983-6_6

2 Antigen-Specific Antibody

Evaluating for antigen-specific IgG antibodies against potential inciting agents of HP is recommended in the practical guideline for diagnosis of HP developed by American Thoracic Society (ATS), Japanese Respiratory Society (JRS), and Asociación Latinoamericana de Tórax (ALAT) in 2020 [1]. Two major methods for the detection of serum antigen-specific IgG are as follows: Ouchterlony double immunodiffusion (DID) and enzyme-linked immunosorbent assay (ELISA). DID has long been used as the basic method, which detects the specific antibodies by formation of a precipitate line that appears between patient serum and antigen applied on the agar gel. Enzyme-linked immunosorbent assay (ELISA) can measure multiple samples quantitatively, and it is more sensitive than DID. ATS/JRS/ALAT guideline reported serum IgG testing against HP-associated antigens distinguishes HP from other ILDs with a sensitivity and specificity of 83% and 68%, respectively, and this decision has been arrived at by pooling data from four studies. A positive serum antigen-specific IgG result does not mean the presence of HP; therefore, diagnosis of HP should be confirmed by further exploring the causative agent in the patients' environment. Additionally, there is no standardized method for evaluating antigen-specific IgG; thus, the guideline committee proposed the development of internationally accepted test as one of the top priorities in this field.

2.1 Bacteria

Saccharopolyspora rectivirgula and *Thermoactinomyces vulgaris*, species of thermophilic bacteria, are identified from moldy hay as the antigens of Farmer‘s lung disease (FLD) by Pepys et al. [2] in 1963. Over the decades, several species of bacteria have been reported as the antigen responsible for occupational and home-related HP. *Mycobacteirum* species, widely distributed in nature and mainly isolated from soil and water, were identified as the antigen responsible for causing hot-tub lung and machine operator's lung (MOL). The latter was caused by *Mycobacterium immunogenum* in contaminated metalworking fluids.

Gram-negative bacteria are also reported as the antigen responsible for causing HP; *Pseudomonas fluorescens* is the antigen responsible for causing MOL, presence of *Pantoea agglomerans* causes wood worker's HP [3], and Species of *Pseudomonas*, *Acinetobacter*, and *Klebiella* are isolated from contaminated water in the humidifier of the patients with humidifier lung [4–6].

Specific IgGs against those bacteria can be detected in the patient's serum. Several reports evaluated the utility of antigen-specific IgG for FLD and MOL patients [7, 8], though there is no internationally standardized method for measuring antigen-specific IgG at present.

Recently, several antigenic components of SR specific for FLD have been identified: glycoproteins of cell wall consist of glucose and mannose, and secretion protease and glycosidase [9, 10]. Specific IgG antibodies against these antigenic components synthesized as recombinant polypeptides have sufficient sensitivity and specificity in preliminary study [9]. Although further studies are required, it is expected to become an international standard method in the future.

Likewise, both acyl-CoA dehydrogenase and dihydrolipoyl dehydrogenase (DLDH) have been identified from *Mycobacterium. immunogenum* (*M.immunogenum*) as the antigenic proteins of MOL [11]. DLDH is also reported as the antigenic component in *Lichtheimia corymbifera* (*L.corymbifera*), one of the fungal species that causes FLD [12]. In patients' sera, specific IgGs against DLDH of unexposed species are detected; DLDH-specific IgGs of *M.immunogenum* in FL and that of *L. corymbifera* in MOL patients, and a correlation is observed between the two [13]. This indicates the cross-reactivity among the antigens of those two species.

2.2 Bird Antigen

Bird antigen is one of the most common causes of HP, and this has been reported from many areas all over the world. The first reported cases in 1960s were caused by breeding birds; so, it has been called bird fanciers' lung or pigeon breeders' lung. However, later it was reported that it is caused by not only direct contact with birds but also by indirect exposure: birds around the home, and the use of feather/ down products such as duvets, down jackets, coats. So, now, it is more appropriate to call as "bird-related hypersensitivity pneumonitis (BRHP)."

Droppings and bloom (feather dust) are the major antigenic sources of BRHP that contain bird serum proteins including immunoglobulins. IgG antibodies against these antigens are present in BRHP patients' serum, though there is no internationally recognized standard test at this point of time. Shirai et al. [14] have demonstrated the clinical utility of the pigeon/parrot/budgerigar-specific IgG with ImmunoCAP® by comparing 75 cases of BRHP (29 acute, 46 chronic: 17 recurrent, 29 insidious), 64 control diseases (15 idiopathic interstitial pneumonias, four idiopathic pulmonary fibrosis, 24 collagen-vascular-disease-related interstitial pneumonia, 10 summer-type hypersensitivity pneumonia, one humidifier lung, 10 other interstitial pneumonias), and 146 healthy volunteers. IgG titers against these three bird species were significantly higher among acute and recurrent types of chronic BRHP patients when compared to the controls (Fig. 6.1). The cutoff values determined are as follows: 24.6 mgA/L for pigeons, 14.0 mgA/L for parrots, and 8.7 mgA/L for parakeets. The sensitivity are 70%, 91%, and 74%; the specificity are 86%, 77%, and 83%, respectively, for acute and recurrent types of chronic BRHP. Moreover, the pigeon−/parrot−/budgerigar-specific IgGs are highly correlated between each other, which indicated the cross-reactivity among bird species, compatible with previous report [15].

On the other hand, among the insidious type of chronic BRHP, a disease phenotype characterized by progressive pulmonary fibrosis, the sensitivities of the pigeon/ parrot/budgerigar-specific IgGs are low, that is, 21%, 45%, and 28%, respectively

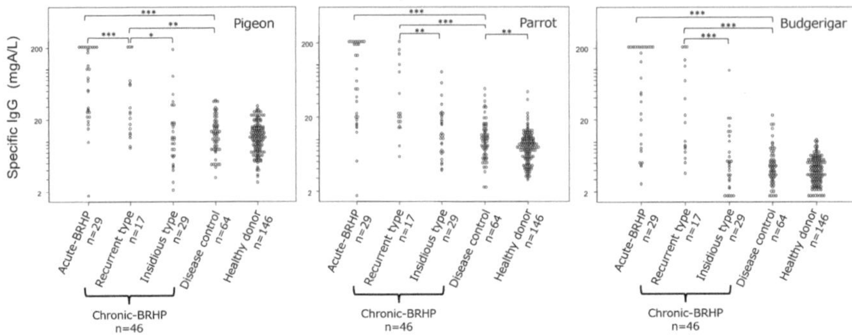

Fig. 6.1 Distribution of bird-specific IgG antibody titers by ImmunoCAP®. Titers determined by ImmunoCAP® of serum IgG against pigeon, parrot, and budgerigar in 75 cases of bird-related hypersensitivity pneumonitis (29 acute, 46 chronic: 17 recurrent-type and 29 insidious-type), 64 disease controls (15 idiopathic interstitial pneumonia, 4 idiopathic pulmonary fibrosis, 24 collagen vascular disease-related interstitial pneumonia, 10 summer-type hypersensitivity pneumonitis, 1 humidifier lung, 10 other interstitial pneumonia), and 146 healthy volunteers. ***: $p < 0.001$, **: $p < 0.01$, *: $p < 0.05$, Mann-Whitney's U Test. *Abbreviations*: BRHP bird-related hypersensitivity pneumonitis. Allergol Int 2021;70:208–214

[14]. This might reflect the difference in the immunopathology between nonfibrotic (acute) and fibrotic (chronic) HP; therefore, the diagnosis of fibrotic HP should be made based on the integration of clinical, radiological, and pathological findings.

Antigenic components in pigeon droppings have been identified: immunoglobulin lambda-like polypeptide-1 (IGLL-1) and proproteinase E (proE) [16, 17]. IGLL-1 is an invariant polypeptide belonging to the immunoglobulin super family, and proproteinase E is a pancreas-secreted zymogen, although in a small number of patients, IgG titers against recombinant IGLL-1 and proE are significantly higher than controls.

2.3 Fungi

Fungi are also common cause of HP, though the causative species differs depending on countries and regions. In Japan, *Trichosporon asahii* (*T. asahii*) and *T. mucoides* are the most well-known fungal antigens of HP, unique molds grow on wood under country-specific house and summer climate condition. Thus, it called summer-type hypersensitivity pneumonitis (SHP).

The major antigenic component of *T. asahii* is identified as the glucuronoxylomannan consisting of 1,3-mannan as the main chain and xylose, mannose, and glucuronic acid as branches with a molecular weight of approximately 800 kD in the capsular polysaccharide. The specific-IgG against this antigen (*T.asahii*-specific IgG) can be measured by antigen-captured ELISA, and values are indicated as corrected absorbance index (CAI) that is calculated by the absorbance of the sample and positive control. The sensitivity and specificity of *T.asahii*-specific IgG were

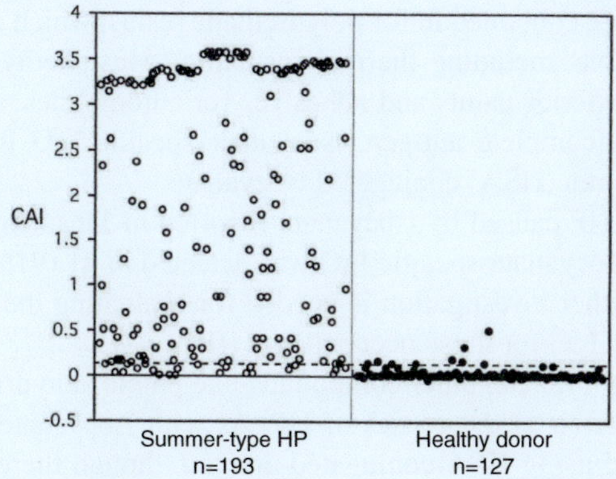

Fig. 6.2 Distribution of *Trichosporon asahii*-specific IgG antibody titer by antigen-captured ELISA. Titers determined by antigen-captured ELISA of serum IgG against *Trichosporon asahii* in 193 cases of summer-type hypersensitivity pneumonitis and 127 healthy volunteers. *Abbreviations*: CAI corrected absorbance index, ELISA enzyme-linked immunosorbent assay. Journal of the Japan Respiratory Society 2001;39:7

87% and 96% when the cutoff is set to 0.15 CAI, calculated by comparing 193 SHP patients and 127 healthy subjects (Fig. 6.2) [18].

In Europe, fungi are known as one of the common antigens of FLD other than thermophilic actinomycetes. *Aspergillus* are considered as a common causative species of FLD based on the studies evaluating the presence of fungal-specific IgGs in the serum of FLD patients [19, 20]. Both in the East of French and Finland, *Lichtheimia corymbifera* (*L. corymbifera*) is reported to be another common cause of FLD: levels of serum IgG antibody against *L. corymbifera* are significantly higher in the FLD patients than control farmers [21, 22].

Several species of *Penicllium* are identified as the antigen of occupational HP, including food industry workers; peat moss processing [23], onion and potato sorter [24], dry sausage/ salami brushing [25, 26], cheese washer [27], cork workers [28], construction plasterer handling esparto fibres [29] and also reported HP caused by the equipment in their home or office; camper [30], humidifier [31], fuel chip [32] and so on. In these cases, *Penicillium*-specific IgG was detected in patients' serum, though methods employed are different in each of these cases. Some laboratories provided the commercially available IgG panel for HP including common fungi and thermos actinomycetes as antigen.

2.4 Chemicals

Some of the chemicals used in industries are reported as antigen of occupational HP. Isocyanates are one of the major low-molecular-weight compounds that cause HP: toluene diisocyanate (TDI), methylenediphenyl diisocyanate (MDI), and hexamethylene diisocyanate (HDI).

TDI and MDI are contained in for polyurethane resins, which are used in a wide range of applications including thermal insulation. Hexamethylene diisocyanate (HDI) is used in exterior paints and adhesives for automobiles and aircraft. Since isocyanate is an incomplete antigen, isocyanate-specific IgG is measured using human serum albumin (HSA) conjugated isocyanate.

In the cases of HP caused by isocyanate reported in Japan from 1982 to 2006, HSA-conjugated isocyanate-specific IgG was detected in 21 (91%) out of 23 cases [33]. However, further investigation is needed for evaluating the clinical utility of isocyanate-specific IgG for those occupational HP.

In addition to isocyanate, other compounds like phthic anhydride and trimellitic anhydride are reported as the causes of HP. As with isocyanate, antigen-specific IgGs are measured using HSA-conjugated antigen, though there are no commercially available tests for this.

2.5 *Individualized Approach*

Although a number of bacterial and fungal species could act as the antigen for HP, the number of antigens commercially available for antigen-specific IgG is quite limited. To overcome this dilemma, individual approach has been proposed that uses antigens collected in the environment of individual HP patients [34]. Specific IgG antibodies can be detected by this method when the commercial panel test was negative. However, this "patient-centered" assessment is not commercially available, and is performed only in centers with research facilities.

3 Lymphocyte Proliferation Test

Lymphocyte proliferation test (LPT), also called as lymphocyte-stimulating test (LST), is a method that evaluates the presence of antigen-sensitized T lymphocytes by stimulating peripheral blood mononuclear cells (PBMCs) or bronchoalveolar lavage (BALF) lymphocytes with suspicious antigen. Specifically, PBMCs or BALF lymphocytes are incubated with suspected antigen, and then H^3-thymidine is added, cell proliferation is evaluated by the amount of H^3-thymidine uptake measured with a scintillation counter. The ratio of the unstimulated sample to the sample stimulated with antigen is expressed as stimulation index (S.I).

Although the 2020 ATS/JRS/ALAT HP guideline did not refer LPT, ATS workshop on exposure assessment tools for HP, held on 2019, described LPT [35]. According to the workshop repot, LPT is expected as an exposure assessment tool especially for the patients who do not exhibit serum-specific IgG antibodies to the inciting antigen, though there are obstacles for use in clinical practice: there is no standardized method or guidance for what constitutes a positive test result, and most studies that report the utility of LPT have examined only those patients with HP suspected to be caused by bird's antigen.

Table 6.1 Sensitivity and specificity of the lymphocyte proliferation test with pigeon plasma of bird-related hypersensitivity pneumonitis

Disease type	Sample	Cutoff value (S.I.)	Sensitivity (%)	Specificity (%)
Acute	PBMCs	2.48	50	100
	BALF lymphocytes	1.55	100	100
Chronic	PBMCs	2.01	46	91
	BALF lymphocytes	NA	NA	NA

S.I. stimulation index, *NA* not available

Suhara et al. [36] have investigated the clinical utility of LPT cultured with pigeon sera for the diagnosis of BRHP by comparing 45 cases of BRHP (10 acute, 35 chronic), 14 SHP, and 76 other interstitial lung diseases. In this report, the sensitivity and specificity of LPT for acute and chronic BRHP were evaluated separately. In the acute BRHP patients, the sensitivity and specificity were 50% and 100% on PBMCs, but 100% and 100% on BALF lymphocytes. In contrast, in the chronic BRHP patients, the sensitivity and specificity of LPT performed on PBMCs were 46% and 91%, respectively. The sensitivity and specificity of LPT in acute and chronic BRHP are summarized in Table 6.1.

Furthermore, Ohtani et al. [37] reported positive rates of antigen-specific IgG and LPT of 32 patients with chronic BRHP evaluated by the type of the chronic HP: recurrent and insidious. Recurrent type is characterized by repeated acute episodes with pulmonary fibrosis as chronic inflammation. Insidious type is the same as the fibrotic HP, which is characterized by progressive pulmonary fibrosis. While the positive rates of antigen-specific IgG among these two types were different, 86% in the recurrent type and 35% in the insidious type, LPT was positive with over 90% in both types of the disease.

According to these results, LPT has a potential to be a supplemental tool for the diagnosis and antigen identification of HP. However, currently, there is no standardized protocol, and further investigation is needed to evaluate clinical utility of LPT for other than bird antigens.

4 Conclusion

Immunological tests for HP are outlined. These tests are clinically important for the diagnosis of HP as well as for the identification of the inciting antigen. Development of internationally accepted test is needed for future clinical investigation.

References

1. Raghu G, Remy-Jardin M, Ryerson CJ, Myers JL, Kreuter M, Vasakova M, Bargagli E, Chung JH, Collins BF, Bendstrup E, et al. Diagnosis of hypersensitivity an official ATS/JRS/ALAT clinical practice guideline. Am J Respir Crit Care Med. 2020;202:e36–69.

2. Pepys J, Jenkins PA, Festenstein GN, Gregory PH, Lacey ME, Skinner FA. Farmer's lung. Thermophilic actinomycetes as a source of "farmer's lung hay" antigen. Lancet. 1963;2(7308):607–11.
3. Mackiewicz B, Dutkiewicz J, Siwiec J, Kucharczyk T, Siek E, Wójcik-Fatla A, Cholewa G, Cholewa A, Paściak M, Pawlik K, Szponar B, Milanowski J. Acute hypersensitivity pneumonitis in woodworkers caused by inhalation of birch dust contaminated with *Pantoea agglomerans* and *Microbacterium barkeri*. Ann Agric Environ Med. 2019;26(4):644–55.
4. Koschel D, Stark W, Karmann F, Sennekamp J, Müller-Wening D. Extrinsic allergic alveolitis caused by misting fountains. Respir Med. 2005;99(8):943–7.
5. Shimoda M, Morimoto K, Tanaka Y, Ken O, Yoshimori K. Humidifier lung induced by endotoxin and various pathogens: characteristic differences from other phenotypes of hypersensitivity pneumonitis. Respir Med Case Rep. 2020;31:101267.
6. Kane GC, Marx JJ, Prince DS. Hypersensitivity pneumonitis secondary to Klebsiella oxytoca. A new cause of humidifier lung. Chest. 1993;104(2):627–9.
7. Ojanen TH, Katila ML, Mäntyjärvi RA. The use of enzyme-linked immunosorbent assay (ELISA) in the diagnosis of farmer's lung. Allergy. 1980;35:537–42.
8. Konishi K, Murakami S, Kokubu K, et al. Determination by enzyme-linked immunosorbent assay (ELISA) of specific IgG antibody activities for diagnosis of farmer's lung disease. Tohoku J Exp Med. 1985;147:135–44.
9. Barrera C, Millon L, Rognon B, et al. Immunoreactive proteins of *Saccharopolyspora rectivirgula* for farmer's lung serodiagnosis. Proteomics Clin Appl. 2014;8:971–81.
10. Mundt C, Becker WM, Schlaak M. Farmer's lung: patients' IgG2 antibodies specifically recognize *Saccharopolyspora rectivirgula* proteins and. J Allergy Clin Immunol. 1996;98:441–50.
11. Roussel S, Rognon B, Barrera C, et al. Immuno-reactive proteins from Mycobacterium immunogenum useful for serodiagnosis of metalworking fluid. Int J Med Microbiol. 2011;301:150–6.
12. Rognon B, Barrera C, Monod M, et al. Identification of antigenic proteins from Lichtheimia corymbifera for farmer's lung disease diagnosis. PLoS One. 2016;11:e0160888.
13. Millon L, Rognon B, Valot B, et al. Common peptide epitopes induce cross-reactivity in hypersensitivity pneumonitis serodiagnosis. J Allergy Clin Immunol. 2016;138:1738–41.
14. Shirai T, Tanino Y, Nikaido T, et al. Screening and diagnosis of acute and chronic bird-related hypersensitivity pneumonitis by serum IgG and IgA antibodies to bird antigens with ImmunoCAP®. Allergol Int. 2021;70:208–14.
15. Sennekamp J, Lange G, Nerger K, Berdel D, Meier-Sydow J. Human antibodies against antigens of the sparrow, blackbird, weaver finch, canary, budgerigar, pigeon and hen using the indirect immunofluorescent technique. Clin Allergy. 1981;11(4):375–84.
16. Shirai T, Furusawa H, Furukawa A, et al. Protein antigen of bird-related hypersensitivity pneumonitis in pigeon serum and dropping. Respir Res. 2017;18:65.
17. Rouzet A, Morell F, Reboux G, et al. Pilot study using recombinant antigens r-PROE and r-IGLL1 for the Serodiagnosis of feather duvet lung. Bronconeumol. 2021;S0300-2896:00073–9.
18. Miyake S, Hamaoka A, Yoshizawa Y. Diagnosis of summer-type hypersensitivity pneumonitis by antigen junction ELISA using mouse anti-Trichosporon asahii monoclonal antibody D-8. J Japan Respir Soc. 2001;39:7.
19. Cano-Jiménez E, Rubal D, Pérez de Llano LA, Mengual N, Castro-Añón O, Méndez L, Golpe R, Sanjuán P, Martín I, Veres A. Farmer's lung disease: analysis of 75 cases. Med Clin (Barc). 2017;149(10):429–35.
20. Sennekamp J, Joest M, Sander I, Engelhart S, Raulf-Heimsoth M. Farmerlungen-Antigene in Deutschland [Farmer's lung antigens in Germany]. Pneumologie. 2012;66(5):297–301.
21. Reboux G, Piarroux R, Mauny F, et al. Role of molds in farmer's lung disease in Eastern France. Am J Respir Crit Care Med. 2001;163:1534–9.
22. Erkinjuntti-Pekkanen R, Reiman M, Kokkarinen JI, Tukiainen HO, Terho EO. IgG antibodies, chronic bronchitis, and pulmonary function values in farmer's lung patients and matched controls. Allergy. 1999;54(11):1181–7.

23. Cormier Y, Israël-Assayag E, Bédard G, Duchaine C. Hypersensitivity pneumonitis in peat moss processing plant workers. Am J Respir Crit Care Med. 1998;158(2):412–7.
24. Merget R, Sander I, Rozynek P, Raulf-Heimsoth M, Bruening T. Occupational hypersensitivity pneumonitis due to molds in an onion and potato sorter. Am J Ind Med. 2008;51(2):117–9.
25. Morell F, Cruz MJ, Gómez FP, Rodriguez-Jerez F, Xaubet A, Muñoz X. Chacinero's lung – hypersensitivity pneumonitis due to dry sausage dust. Scand J Work Environ Health. 2011;37(4):349–56.
26. Marvisi M, Balzarini L, Mancini C, Mouzakiti P. A new type of hypersensitivity pneumonitis: salami brusher's disease. Monaldi Arch Chest Dis. 2012;77(1):35–7.
27. Campbell JA, Kryda MJ, Treuhaft MW, Marx JJ Jr, Roberts RC. Cheese worker's hypersensitivity pneumonitis. Am Rev Respir Dis. 1983;127(4):495–6.
28. Morell F, Roger A, Cruz MJ, Muñoz X, Rodrigo MJ. Suberosis: clinical study and new etiologic agents in a series of eight patients. Chest. 2003;124(3):1145–52.
29. Cruz MJ, Morell F, Roger A, Muñoz X, Rodrigo MJ. Neumonitis por hipersensibilidad en los yeseros de la construcción (espartosis): estudio de 20 casos. Med Clin (Barc). 2003;120(15):578–83.
30. Tiotiu A, Metz-Favre C, Reboux G, Kessler R, de Blay F. Pneumopathie d'hypersensibilité à Penicillium chrysogenum et Streptomyces mésophile: intérêt de l'enquête environnementale à domicile. Rev Pneumol Clin. 2013;69(5):278–82.
31. Solley GO, Hyatt RE. Hypersensitivity pneumonitis induced by Penicillium species. J Allergy Clin Immunol. 1980;65(1):65–70.
32. Van Assendelft AH, Raitio M, Turkia V. Fuel chip-induced hypersensitivity pneumonitis caused by penicillium species. Chest. 1985;87(3):394–6.
33. Tabata H, Mochizuki Y, Nakahara Y, Kobashi Y, Kawamura T, Sasaki S. Hypersensitivity pneumonitis caused by isocyanate exposure during recreational painting. Nihon Kokyuki Gakkai Zasshi. 2009;47(11):1002–7.
34. Millerick-May ML, Mulks MH, Gerlach J, Flaherty KR, Schmidt SL, Martinez FJ, LeVeque RM, Rosenman KD. Hypersensitivity pneumonitis and antigen identification–An alternate approach. Respir Med. 2016;112:97–105.
35. Johannson KA, Barnes H, Bellanger AP, Dalphin JC, Fernández Pérez ER, Flaherty KR, Huang YT, Jones KD, Kawano-Dourado L, Kennedy K, Millerick-May M, Miyazaki Y, Morisset J, Morell F, Raghu GR, Robbins C, Sack CS, Salisbury ML, Selman M, Vasakova M, Walsh SLF, Rose CS. Exposure assessment tools for hypersensitivity pneumonitis. An official American Thoracic Society Workshop Report. Ann Am Thorac Soc. 2020;17:1501–9.
36. Suhara K, Miyazaki Y, Okamoto T, Yasui M, Tsuchiya K, Inase N. Utility of immunological tests for bird-related hypersensitivity pneumonitis. Respir Investig. 2015;53(1):13–21.
37. Ohtani Y, Saiki S, Sumi Y, et al. Clinical features of recurrent and insidious chronic bird fancier's lung. Ann Allergy Asthma Immunol. 2003;90:604–10.

Chapter 7
Exposure Provocation Test and Antigen Avoidance Test

What Are Exposure Provocation Test and Antigen Avoidance Test in Diagnosis of HP?

Ryo Okuda

1 Tests for the Identification of the Inciting Antigen

A very aggressive search will result in the identification of the inciting antigen of fibrotic hypersensitivity pneumonitis (HP) in 40–60% of cases. Questionnaires, specific serum immunoglobulin G (IgG) antibody testing, and the inhalation challenge test have been utilized for the identification and estimation of the inciting antigen; however, these tests have not become the standard method for this task. Serum IgG antibody testing is often used to identify the inciting antigen. However, the accuracy of this method in fibrotic HP is relatively low and a positive serum IgG antibody test result only indicates previous exposure to the inciting antigen. Therefore, a detailed history of exposure is necessary to interpret the test results. However, it is difficult to estimate the degree of exposure based on clinical history-taking, and this approach lacks objectivity. For example, it is not possible to compare the exposure to antigens from maintaining one pigeon in the garden for 20 years with that from maintaining 10 parakeets indoors for 5 years. Identification of the response induced by exposure or avoidance of exposure to the presumed inciting antigen will greatly assist in the diagnosis and identification of the inciting antigen. This chapter describes methods for estimating and identifying the inciting antigen in fibrotic HP, which is a challenging task.

R. Okuda (✉)
Departments of Respiratory Medicine, Kanagawa Cardiovascular and Respiratory Center, Yokohama, Japan
e-mail: okuda.0a20g@kanagawa-pho.jp

Y. Miyazaki (ed.), *Hypersensitivity Pneumonitis*, Respiratory Disease Series: Diagnostic Tools and Disease Managements,
https://doi.org/10.1007/978-981-96-7983-6_7

2 Diagnostic Tests for Fibrotic HP

To improve the diagnostic confidence of fibrotic HP, the main approaches are pathological examination and identification of the inciting antigen. Surgical lung biopsy (SLB) in cases with interstitial lung disease (ILD) may not lead to a definitive diagnosis; 20–30% of all ILDs cases are unclassifiable. Pathology specimens used in SLB may exhibit a usual interstitial pneumonia pattern in cases with long-term exposure to birds, or granulomas and bronchiolocentric fibrosis in cases without obvious history of exposure. The inhalation challenge test and antigen avoidance test can be performed more safely in patients with advanced stage ILD than SLB or transbronchial lung cryobiopsy. Following the diagnosis of fibrotic HP, measures should be recommended for the avoidance of exposure to the inciting antigen.

3 Inhalation Challenge Test

3.1 Avian-Associated Antigens

Pigeon serum, parrot serum, pigeon dropping extract (PDE), pigeon broom (protein attached to feathers), and pigeon eggs have been used (Table 7.1) [1–6]. Pigeon breeder's lung was the first reported case of bird-related HP, and pigeon serum was the first to be used in the inhalation challenge test for this condition. Thus, pigeon is often used as an antigen among avian species. The four methods utilized for pigeon antigen purification are described below.

1. Serum

Serum is most frequently used as an antigen. Pigeon serum is typically collected from the heart of the pigeon using a needle; in some countries, pigeon serum can be purchased. In the 1980s, avian serum was subjects to 5–100-fold dilution prior to usage. However, since the 1990s, blood samples have been sterilized via passage through a filter (pore size: 0.22 μm); subsequently, inhalation is performed by diluting the samples with saline to a concentration of 3 mg protein/mL after boiling at 56 °C for 30 min to inactivate the complement.

2. Feathers

Bloom extraction from feather fragments is conducted using a Soxhlet apparatus, and involves dewaxing with anhydrous ether, dissolution in ammonium bicarbonate water, and centrifugation. The supernatant is dialyzed until a clear extract is obtained, which is lyophilized and stored for dissolution upon inhalation.

3. PDE

PDE is dissolved in phosphate-buffered saline, treated with ammonium sulfate, thoroughly dialyzed, and lyophilized to obtain partially purified PDE. The

Table 7.1 Summary of inhalation challenge tests

	Subjects	Control	Antigens	Items with significant differences	Items without significant differences
Hendrick	Acute or fibrotic HP: 18 cases (bird related: 15, fungus related: 3)	Healthy volunteer: 2	Serum or PDE	Body temperature, FVC, PaO_2, and SaO_2	Shortness of breath, DLco, lymphocyte and neutrophil counts in peripheral blood
Ramirez-Venegas	Bird-related fibrotic HP: 17 cases	Other ILDs: 17, healthy volunteers: 5	Serum	Not applicable	Not applicable
Morell	Bird-related acute HP: 32, subacute: 37, fibrotic: 15 cases	Other ILDs: 20, healthy volunteers: 20	Serum and bloom	Not applicable	Not applicable
Ohtani	Bird-related fibrotic HP: 11 cases	IPF: 2, bird breeders: 4	PDE	Shortness of breath, temperature, A-aDO_2, white blood cell count	VC, DLco, CRP
Ishizuka	Bird-related fibrotic HP: 28 cases	Other ILDs: 19	PDE	White blood cell counts, A-aDO_2	Body temperature, symptoms, VC, DLco
Okuda	Bird-related fibrotic HP: 19 cases	IPF: 5, unidentified fibrotic HP: 12	Egg	FVC, A-aDO_2, CRP, erythrocyte sedimentation rate, LDH, CT findings	Body temperature, white blood cell count, PaO_2

supernatant of the PDE solution (2 mL), adjusted to a protein concentration of 340 μg/mL, is inhaled.

4. Eggs

The egg surface is washed with a sodium hypochlorite solution of ≥150 ppm, pasteurized twice, diluted with saline solution, and inhaled.

3.2 Fungi and Bacteria

The causative fungi vary widely between countries and geographical regions. In Japan, acute (summer) HP caused by *Trichosporon* spp. is common, and inhalation challenge testing for this agent is frequently reported. In Spain and the United States of America, *Penicillium* spp. (*Penicillium frequentans*), *Aspergillus* spp. (*Aspergillus fumigatus*), and *Mucor* spp. (*Mucor mucedo*) are linked to HP, and inhalation is performed at antigen concentrations of 0.01–0.1 mg/mL. Moreover, *Penicillium* spp. has been found in cork. For the identification of fungi, extraction liquid is used in all cases. If HP due to devices (e.g., humidifiers or air conditioners) is suspected, the suspect devices are used in the patient's room or home, and confirm the immunological reaction. Bacteria are rarely used as inhalation challenging material because of the endotoxin. Humidifier lung caused by bacteria exhibits higher inflammatory indices, such as white blood cells (WBC) and C-reactive protein (CRP), more infiltrative shadows on high-resolution computed tomography (HRCT), and elevated neutrophils and fewer lymphocytes in bronchial alveolar lavage fluid compared with acute HP caused by fungi. These differences are attributed to endotoxin.

4 Methods of Inhalation Challenge Test

Inhalation should be performed for 2–20 min and 15–30 min with a jet nebulizer and an ultrasonic nebulizer, respectively. In the absence of an apparent response after 24 h of inhalation, a second inhalation test can be performed the next day at the same concentration or 24–48 h later at a ten-fold higher inhalation concentration. Alternatively, the antigen concentration can be increased stepwise (5–10-fold increase). Inhalation can be performed in a private room in a hospital and followed up under inpatient or outpatient care. The use of a small room allows investigators to limit the exposure to the antigen to 5–20 min of inhalation time. This approach avoids exposure of the patient and health-care professionals after completion of the inhalation.

4.1 Main Parameters

Body temperature measurement, respiratory function testing, blood testing, arterial blood gas analysis, and HRCT findings are used for evaluation. Body temperature is often measured every hour from the initiation of inhalation until 24 h later; forced vital capacity (FVC) and diffusing capacity of lung for carbon monoxide (DLco) are measured before testing and twice thereafter (at 6 h and 24 h). A portable pulmonary function test is also used to measure FVC every hour. Blood samples are obtained before the test and at 6–8 h and 24 h later. Analysis of partial pressure of arterial oxygen (PaO_2), partial pressure of arterial carbon dioxide ($PaCO_2$), leukocytes, leukocyte fractions, erythrocyte sedimentation rate (ESR), and CRP is performed. Interstitial pneumonia markers, such as Krebs von den Lungen-6 (KL-6) and surfactant protein-D and anti-pigeon IgG antibody titer, are not indicators. Chest X-ray examination may be performed after 24 h; however, HRCT may be an option, because it is not possible to discern subtle changes via X-ray analysis.

4.2 Positive Criteria

Since the magnitude of the response depends on the type and concentration of antigen used, it is important to compare the change after inhalation with control. Inhalation of distilled water can also be used as a placebo for comparison with the solution containing the purified antigen. The following information is a guideline for determining the positivity of each item based on previous reports.

4.3 Important Items

Body temperature: elevation by 0.5–1.0 °C or higher
WBC: elevation by 20–30% or more
CRP: elevation by 0.3–1 mg/dL or more
Alveolar-arterial oxygen difference (A-aDO_2): >10 Torr

4.4 Supplemental Items

PaO_2: decrease by 3–10 Torr or more
Peripheral oxygen saturation (SpO_2): decrease of 3% or more
ESR: elevation by >2 mm/1 h
FVC: decrease by 10–15% or more
DLco: decrease by >20%
HRCT: increase in frosted shadows in the upper lobe or worsening of reticular or frosted shadows around existing interstitial shadows
Symptoms: worsening of dyspnea and cough

4.5 Other Endpoints

Increase in neutrophils, decrease in lymphocytes, respiratory frequency in the exercise stress test. The inhalation provocation test prediction score = 1 × Δ WBC (%) + 2 × Δ A-aDO_2 (Torr) with a cutoff value of 35 has been proposed, and the judgment is centered on leukocytes and A-aDO_2. Since PaO_2 is greatly influenced by the respiratory rate, A-aDO_2 is a more reliable parameter. In other countries, the criteria are based mainly on %FVC, WBC, and PaO_2. For example, a relatively large %FVC decrease of 10–15% may be the criterion, because inhalation challenge testing is performed without distinguishing between cases with nonfibrotic and fibrotic HP. However, in a study, the average FVC decline in the positive inhalation challenge group was 8%, and a decline in DLco by ≥15% was observed in two of 12 cases. Additionally, an inhalation challenge test for fibrotic HP showed a decline in %FVC by 0.5–2%. Further investigation is warranted to determine the threshold for the respiratory function test and its contribution to the diagnosis (Table 7.2). Exacerbation of symptoms can be caused by immunological reactions and irritation from inhalation. Therefore, it is important to compare the results with those of control and placebo inhalation. Most of the above criteria were established for the diagnosis of nonfibrotic and fibrotic bird-related HP; the same criteria were used for

Table 7.2 Mean changes in positive inhalation challenge tests

	Subjects	Temperature	FVC	DLco	PaO_2	A-aDO_2	WBC counts	CRP (mg/dL)
Hendrick	Acute or fibrotic HP: 18 (bird related: 15, fungus related: 3)	1.4 °C	−20%, −610 mL	n/a	n/a	n/a	n/a	n/a
Ramirez-Venegas	Bird-related fibrotic HP: 17 cases	2.5 °C	−361 mL	n/a	−8 Torr	n/a	−2198/μL	n/a
Ohtani	Bird-related fibrotic HP: 11 cases	1.1 °C	−0.6%	−8.1%	n/a	10.8 Torr	61%	1.4
Ishizuka	Bird-related fibrotic HP: 28 cases	1.0 °C	−2.3%	−5.8%	n/a	7.9 Torr	63%	1.0
Okuda	Bird-related fibrotic HP: 19 cases	0.1 °C	−1.1%	n/a	−8 Torr	6.3 Torr	15%	0.3

fungal extracts. However, further study is required, because the types of antigens and degree of exposure differ. In inhalation challenge testing with devices, such as humidifiers and air conditioners, it is difficult to identify a single antigen, because multiple bacteria and fungi are often identified by the device. Nevertheless, this kind of testing is useful for the identification of the causative device.

4.6 *Eligibility Criteria*

Cases of suspected HP, including fibrotic HP, are eligible. Cases with the following characteristics should be carefully examined:

1. Difficulty in performing a respiratory function test.
2. FVC <50% and DLco <40%.
3. $PaO_2 < 60$ Torr.

However, it has been reported that the inhalation challenge test can be safely performed even in patients with a $PaO_2 < 60$ Torr. In cases with elevated inflammatory factors, such as WBC and CRP, the patients should be hospitalized for adequate antigen avoidance. Moreover, the test should be performed after the patient's condition has stabilized. If possible, the administration of anti-inflammatory drugs (e.g., prednisolone and immunosuppressive agents) should be discontinued 1 week prior to inhalation. If this is not possible, physicians should consider reducing the dose of these drugs prior to testing.

4.7 Position in the Guidelines

1. In the 2021 CHEST Diagnosis and Evaluation of HP guidelines, it is weakly recommended not to perform inhalation challenge test due to unstandardized testing and insufficient validation of positive criteria [7].
2. In the HP Diagnostic Guidelines of the American Thoracic Society, Japanese Respiratory Society, and Latin American Thoracic Association published in 2020 [8], the inhalation challenge test is not well described. It is only stated that the inhalation challenge test should be performed at facilities with experience in this field. Regarding antigen-specific testing, anti-IgG antibodies are mainly described. It has been reported that the sensitivity and specificity of serum IgG antibody testing are 83% and 68%, respectively. Serum IgG antibody testing is rated as a convenient and sufficiently generalized method. However, it has been judged to be inferior to the questionnaire for the diagnosis or exclusion of HP. It is also cautioned that positivity for IgG antibody does not indicate the HP-causing antigen. Instead, it only confirms prior exposure of the patient to the HP-causing antigen.
3. In the diagnostic criteria for chronic HP published in 2018 (modified Delphi Survey) [9], 45 ILD specialists from 14 countries selected 49 laboratory findings of high importance for the diagnosis of chronic HP. History of exposure to the HP-causing antigen, mosaic findings on HRCT, nonnecrotizing granulomas, and improvement with antigen avoidance were selected as important items. The inhalation challenge test, lymphocyte proliferation test, and precipitating antibodies were selected among those 49 items; however, these were not considered the most important tests. Currently, the usefulness of the inhalation challenge test is reduced by the insufficient data, nonstandardization of testing methods, and its limited availability in clinics.

4.8 Safety

The inhalation challenge test for chronic HP (fibrotic HP) may induce acute exacerbation and progression of the underlying disease. Ohtani and Ishizuka et al. suggested that the inhalation challenge test should not be performed in cases with $PaO_2 < 60$ Torr, and they also suggested that cases with elevated inflammatory responses, such as CRP and WBC, should be hospitalized to ensure adequate avoidance of antigens [4, 5]. The inhalation challenge test should be conducted only when the patient's condition becomes stable. Munoz and Morell et al. did not observe immediate reactions (e.g., bronchoconstriction or wheezing) in 39 patients who underwent the inhalation challenge test; the decline in FVC induced by testing improved after 3 months [10].

As a rule, the inhalation challenge test was not performed in any of the following cases:

1. Patients with myocardial infarction or cerebrovascular disease (within 3 months), serious arrhythmia, poorly controlled epileptic seizure, or lack of a respiratory function test
2. Patients for whom pulmonary function tests were not performed
3. Patients with FVC <50% or DLco <40%
4. Patients with $PaO_2 < 60$ Torr

Based on previous reports, we did not perform inhalation challenge test in patients with FVC <50% or $PaO_2 < 60$ Torr.

There were no early immunological reactions observed in patients with positivity for specific IgE antibodies against PDE when the inhalation test was performed using pigeon serum. A skin prick test may also be performed to identify patients exhibiting immediate immunological reactions.

5 Common Antigens

In 130 cases in the HP and control groups combined, the correlation between serum IgG antibody titers of pigeons, parrots, and parakeets was very high, ranging from 0.92 to 0.97 [11]. In addition, even in fungi that are taxonomically very far apart, there is a high degree of structural homology and common allergens have been demonstrated. Thus, immune responses may occur to a wide variety of fungi, and the inciting fungus of fibrotic HP may not be identifiable.

6 Natural Provocation Test (Environmental Exposure Test)

Uzun et al. performed a natural provocation test on eight cases of bird-related acute HP; the test was positive for one of those cases [12]. The approach included X-ray examination, pulmonary function testing, and blood sampling at 8:00 a.m. for cases with few symptoms. This was followed by contact with pigeons (shed cleaning, feeding) as usual, and return to the hospital 8 h later to perform the test.

A positive result is based on the presence of three or more of the following items:

1. Increased abnormal shadows on X-ray analysis
2. Δ A-aDO_2 opening >10 Torr or decrease in DLco by >20%
3. Decline in vital capacity (VC) by >15%
4. Increase in peripheral blood lymphocytes by >30%
5. Increase in CRP by >1 mg/dL
6. Increase in body temperature by >1 °C or appearance of systemic symptoms, such as chills and fatigue
7. Appearance of respiratory symptoms, such as cough and shortness of breath

The natural provocation test, performed on one case of chronic bird-related HP, was negative. Because acute HP is easily diagnosed through the antigen avoidance test, the natural provocation test is rarely performed to diagnose acute bird-related HP. In addition, it is difficult to standardize the natural provocation test, because the degree of exposure varies greatly depending on the living environment of the patient. The natural provocation test was not mentioned in the 2021 CHEST Diagnosis and Evaluation of HP guidelines or in the 2018 modified Delphi survey. In clinical practice, inpatients with nonfibrotic HP or acute on chronic (fibrotic) HP may be requested to return to the clinic a few hours or days later for the natural provocation test. However, robust criteria and conclusions on the duration of exposure for testing have not been established thus far. Furthermore, the degree of exposure during the natural provocation test also varies between cases; hence, defining a constant duration of exposure for all cases may not be useful.

7 Antigen Avoidance Test

Firstly, antigen avoidance refers to the removal of the inciting antigen for HP from the living environment of the patient. The use of antigen avoidance as a test (tool) is valuable, because the evaluation of response may have both diagnostic and prognostic implications. The diagnosis and treatment of nonfibrotic (acute) HP is easier, because the condition clearly and rapidly improves following antigen avoidance alone. Thus, an "antigen avoidance test" is not essential.

The types of inciting antigens are diverse and vary widely between geographical regions. However, environmental fungi and birds are the most frequent inciting antigens for fibrotic HP. Antigen avoidance includes cleaning and relocation to a new home or workplace, changing employment, discontinuation of bird keeping, and disposal of feather products and humidifiers. These measures are useful in cases with a diagnosis of fibrotic HP and clear identification of a single inciting antigen. Nevertheless, in numerous cases with fibrotic HP, the diagnosis is not definitive. Consequently, patients are often misdiagnosed with idiopathic pulmonary fibrosis or other interstitial lung diseases. In addition, clinical history-taking and/or specific serum IgG antibody testing alone cannot identify a single inciting antigen. Nonfibrotic HP, acute on fibrotic HP, or acute exacerbation of fibrotic HP should be suspected in cases in which a single inciting antigen can be identified from a clinical history-taking and/or specific serum IgG antibody testing. In cases of fibrotic HP in which fibrosis has already progressed, short-term antigen avoidance is not curative; however, changes in parameters resulting from strict short-term antigen avoidance may be of high value in the diagnostic process for fibrotic HP. Antigen avoidance may be performed as a "test" for the diagnosis and identification of the inciting antigen. Apart from its diagnostic value, the identification of the inciting antigen also affects the outcome of fibrotic HP.

Numerous reported have stated that sustained antigen avoidance improves the prognosis of fibrotic HP. However, thus far, there are few reports on the use of the antigen avoidance test for diagnosis, although the short-term antigen avoidance test requires a positive or negative criterion. The antigen avoidance test involves a 14-day hospitalization to isolate the patient from the home or work environment and to compare changes in various parameters for fibrotic HP before and after hospitalization [13]. During hospitalization, patients are not allowed to leave the hospital or use down quilts; if a 14-day hospitalization is not possible, patients may be asked to live away from home (e.g., hotel, sibling's house, vacation home, etc.). Evaluation after antigen avoidance should include improvement of symptoms (e.g., shortness of breath, cough, fever, appetite, weight, and fatigue), pulmonary function test, chest X-ray examination, chest HRCT, interstitial pneumonia markers (e.g., KL-6), arterial blood gas analysis, CRP, ESR, total cell count in bronchoalveolar lavage fluid, and antigen levels at home as indicators.

The average changes over a 14-day hospitalization in 196 cases with chronic HP included an increase in VC by 60 mL, a decline in KL-6 by 180 U/mL, a decline in surfactant protein-D by 30 ng/mL, a decline in leukocytes by 770/μL, an improvement in CRP by 0.15 mg/dL, an improvement in A-aDO$_2$ by 3 mmHg, and a decline in body temperature by 0.1 °C (Table 7.3). The criteria for positivity were as follows: improvement in VC by ≥2.5%; improvement in KL-6 and WBC counts by ≥12% and ≥2.5%, respectively; and improvement in at least two of VC, KL-6, and WBC; the reported sensitivity and specificity rates were 51% and 81%, respectively [13]. A shortcoming of these criteria is the low cutoff values used for each parameter. In particular, a 2.5% improvement in WBC counts may be less than a clinically important minimal change. The change in temperature was considered less than a clinically important minimal change and was thus excluded from the criteria. HRCT can easily determine changes induced by antigen avoidance. However, HRCT findings lack objectivity, because this examination is based on visual judgment. Moreover, it is difficult to perform quantitative analysis on each case in clinical practice due to the lack of standardized analysis methods and time. The control group cases used to set these thresholds comprised cases of suspected chronic (fibrotic) HP that were eventually diagnosed with ILD other than HP; therefore, a bias exists in the control group. However, in the positive group (n = 17) for the antigen avoidance test, patients were judged according to these criteria by family members who improved the environment in and around their homes during the antigen avoidance test. The patients showed a −6.5% and −0.3% change in FVC during the year before the test in the positive (n = 17) and

Table 7.3 Changes during 14-day antigen avoidance test

Parameters	Chronic HP (n = 196)	P values
Δ VC, L	0.06 ± 0.01	<0.001
Δ KL-6, U/mL	−182 ± 32	<0.001
Δ SP-D, ng/mL	−30 ± 9	<0.001
Δ WBC, /μL	−771 ± 114	<0.001
Δ CRP, mg/dL	−0.15 ± 0.04	<0.01
Δ A-aDO$_2$, mmHg	−3.3 ± 0.7	<0.001
Δ Body temperature, °C	−0.12 ± 0.02	<0.001

negative ($n = 23$) groups, respectively. The FVC change in the following year was better in the positive group versus the negative group (+0.8% vs. −5.0%, respectively). Multivariate analysis showed that antigen avoidance test results were associated with the prognosis or development of acute exacerbation [14]. Of note, some cases refused to be isolated in the hospital for 2 weeks. Moreover, a few patients were initially admitted but subsequently requested early discharge due to boredom. In addition, a positive antigen avoidance test does not lead to single-antigen identification; it only suggests the presence of inciting antigens in the living environment of the patients. Furthermore, if disease progression is observed, the possibility of persistent exposure to the inciting antigen should be considered even after the antigen avoidance test.

The 2021 CHEST Diagnosis and Evaluation of HP guidelines describe the interpretation of the antigen avoidance test as follows [7]. Clinically important improvement in symptoms, as well as physiological and radiological features, may be observed only in patients with nonfibrotic HP. Measurable clinical improvement may not occur in patients in whom the improved antigen was not the inciting antigen causing HP, who have multiple disease-inciting exposures, for whom complete antigen avoidance cannot be achieved, or those with severe or progressive pulmonary fibrosis. Furthermore, inciting antigens may not be identified in patients with severe pulmonary fibrosis. Thus, clinical improvement following antigen avoidance may support the diagnosis of HP; however, the lack of clinical improvement does not rule out the possibility of HP.

8 After Antigen Identification Testing

After testing, patients may be asked to improve or avoid their home or work environment or to dispose of feather products or pets. Although these measures are effective against disease progression, the patient's financial barriers and attachment to the source of the inciting antigen may prevent them from implementing effective antigen avoidance. Also, if antigen avoidance is implemented, it may significantly compromise the beliefs of patients and their emotional attachment to pets and hobbies. Of note, despite implementation of these antigen avoidance measures, exposure to the antigen remains possible.

9 Future Issues

Unstandardized testing and the lack of sensitivity remain important challenges for both the inhalation challenge and antigen avoidance tests. The geographical region in which a patient resides should be taken into account to improve the accuracy of these tests.

References

1. Hendrick DJ, Marshall R, Faux JA, Krall JM. Positive "alveolar" responses to antigen inhalation provocation tests: their validity and recognition. Thorax. 1980;35(6):415–27.
2. Ramirez-Venegas A, Sansores RH, Perez-Padilla R, Carrillo G, Selman M. Utility of a provocation test for diagnosis of chronic pigeon Breeder's disease. Am J Respir Crit Care Med. 1998;158(3):862–9.
3. Morell F, Roger A, Reyes L, Cruz MJ, Murio C, Munoz X. Bird fancier's lung: a series of 86 patients. Medicine (Baltimore). 2008;87(2):110–30.
4. Ohtani Y, Kojima K, Sumi Y, Sawada M, Inase N, Miyake S, et al. Inhalation provocation tests in chronic bird fancier's lung. Chest. 2000;118(5):1382–9.
5. Ishizuka M, Miyazaki Y, Tateishi T, Tsutsui T, Tsuchiya K, Inase N. Validation of inhalation provocation test in chronic bird-related hypersensitivity pneumonitis and new prediction score. Ann Am Thorac Soc. 2015;12(2):167–73.
6. Okuda R, Takemura T, Mikami Y, Hagiwara E, Iwasawa T, Baba T, et al. Inhalation challenge test using pigeon eggs for chronic hypersensitivity pneumonitis. Clin Exp Allergy. 2020;50(12):1381–90.
7. Fernandez Perez ER, Travis WD, Lynch DA, Brown KK, Johannson KA, Selman M, et al. Executive summary diagnosis and evaluation of hypersensitivity pneumonitis: CHEST guideline and expert panel report. Chest. 2021;160:e97.
8. Raghu G, Remy-Jardin M, Ryerson CJ, Myers JL, Kreuter M, Vasakova M, et al. Diagnosis of hypersensitivity pneumonitis in adults. An official ATS/JRS/ALAT clinical practice guideline. Am J Respir Crit Care Med. 2020;202(3):e36–69.
9. Morisset J, Johannson KA, Jones KD, Wolters PJ, Collard HR, Walsh SLF, et al. Identification of diagnostic criteria for chronic hypersensitivity pneumonitis: an international modified Delphi survey. Am J Respir Crit Care Med. 2018;197(8):1036–44.
10. Munoz X, Morell F, Cruz MJ. The use of specific inhalation challenge in hypersensitivity pneumonitis. Curr Opin Allergy Clin Immunol. 2013;13(2):151–8.
11. Shirai T, Tanino Y, Nikaido T, Takaku Y, Hashimoto S, Taguchi Y, et al. Screening and diagnosis of acute and chronic bird-related hypersensitivity pneumonitis by serum IgG and IgA antibodies to bird antigens with ImmunoCAP(R). Allergol Int. 2021;70(2):208–14.
12. Uzun O, Yilmaz DK, Sunter AT, Erkan L. The prevalence of "pigeon breeder's disease" in a Turkish city and review of the literature. Lung. 2011;189(3):243–50.
13. Tsutsui T, Miyazaki Y, Okamoto T, Tateishi T, Furusawa H, Tsuchiya K, et al. Antigen avoidance tests for diagnosis of chronic hypersensitivity pneumonitis. Respir Investig. 2015;53(5):217–24.
14. Okuda R, Takemura T, Iwasawa T, Kaburaki S, Baba T, Hagiwara E, et al. Impact of antigen avoidance test for fibrotic hypersensitivity pneumonitis in stable phase. Allergy Asthma Clin Immunol. 2022;18(1):104.

Chapter 8
Biomarker

What Are Biomarkers in Diagnosis of HP?

Haruhiko Furusawa

1 Introduction

Currently, there is no specific serum biomarker for the diagnosis of hypersensitivity pneumonitis (HP), and a comprehensive diagnosis is based on the clinical course, antigen exposure history, and radiological and pathological findings. Proteins and cytokines involved in alveolar injury and inflammation have been investigated as biomarkers for HP. Krebs von den Lungen-6 (KL-6), lung surface-activated protein D (SP-D), and surfactant protein A (SP-A), although not specific to HP, have been reported as potential biomarkers for HP. The seasonal fluctuation of these markers might be reflecting antigen exposure, which is suggestive of HP. In addition, many inflammation markers including CXCR3, CXCL9, and periostin are expected to be candidates for biomarkers in the future. This chapter outlines the characteristics and interpretation of these biomarkers in HP.

2 KL-6 and SP-D

KL-6 is a transmembrane nonsecreted mucin MUC1 glycoprotein with a molecular weight of over 1000 KDa and a total length of 200–500 nm, and is expressed on the lumenal side of type II alveolar epithelial cells, bronchial epithelial cells, and pancreatic and mammary epithelial cells. In interstitial lung diseases including HP, KL-6 is released into blood with alveolar and capillary permeability caused by alveolar epithelial injury

H. Furusawa (✉)
The Department of Respiratory Medicine, Institute of Science Tokyo,
Tokyo, Japan
e-mail: hfurusawa.pulm@tmd.ac.jp

Y. Miyazaki (ed.), *Hypersensitivity Pneumonitis*, Respiratory Disease Series: Diagnostic Tools and Disease Managements,
https://doi.org/10.1007/978-981-96-7983-6_8

[1]. The alveolar epithelial injury also promotes the overexpression of KL-6 by type II alveolar epithelial cell proliferation to cover the injured epithelium, resulting in the elevation of KL-6 in serum and bronchoalveolar lavage fluid [2]. SP-D is a secreted glycoprotein belonging to the collectin family and is produced and secreted by type II alveolar epithelial cells and club cells in the lungs. Its multimeric molecular weight is approximately 500 kDa and its molecular diameter is 90–100 nm, smaller than KL-6, and it is excreted into the blood by alveolar epithelial injury as well as KL-6. Serum KL-6 and SP-D are elevated in many types of HP, including summer-type HP, mushroom grower's lung, farmer's lung, and bird-related HP [3–10], and BALF lymphocyte count correlates with serum KL-6 and SP-D [1, 6, 8, 11]. Seasonal variation in KL-6 and SP-D is a valuable diagnostic marker for HP; since KL-6 and SP-D increase with antigen exposure and decrease with antigen avoidance, an increase during winter may indicate bird-related HP associated with feather products, while an increase during the rainy season or summer may indicate summer-type HP affected by fungus [10–13]. Seasonal variation in the ratio of maximum to minimum serum KL-6 values greater than 3.15-fold is highly suggestive of HP (AUC 0.757, sensitivity 66.7%, specificity 76.9%), especially if the maximum winter KL-6 value is more than 1.64-fold higher than the maximum summer value (AUC 0.878, sensitivity 77.8%, specificity 92.7%) [12].

A decrease in serum KL-6 due to antigen avoidance is also valuable for diagnosis, monitoring, and prognostic estimation [8, 11, 12, 14, 15]. There are several criteria for diagnosing HP from other ILDs. Two-week hospitalization for antigen avoidance with at least two of the following criteria is diagnostic for chronic HP: (1) an increase in FVC of at least 3%, (2) a decrease in KL-6 of at least 13%, or (3) a decrease in white blood cell count of at least 3%. The sensitivity and specificity are 51.0% and 80.7%, respectively [14], and prognosis is poor when KL-6 decreases by less than 10% [15]. In another study, chronic summer-type HP was differentiated from IPF when all of the following criteria are met: (1) positive *Trichosporon asahii* antibody, (2) mosaic pattern or micronodules in chest high-resolution CT (HRCT), and (3) KL-6 > 1500 U/mL or SP-D > 250 ng/mL (AUC 0.965) [16].

In acute HP, KL-6 is markedly elevated and seasonal variation is greater than that in other ILD or chronic HPs, which may reflect an increase in regenerative type II epithelial cells [12, 17]. Drug-induced pneumonia in the HP pattern with diffuse ground grass attenuation often does not elevate serum KL-6 at diagnosis, which may be useful in differentiating it from acute HP [18]. Serum KL-6 did not increase in some cases of humidifier lung in which lung injury is evoked by endotoxin and does not involve an allergic mechanism [19]. KL-6 is also elevated in several types of carcinomas, including non-small cell lung carcinoma, breast cancer, pancreatic cancer, and ovarian cancer, and should be noted for these diseases other than ILD.

3 Th1, Th2, and Th17 Cytokines

Acute HP is mainly caused by Th1 and Th17 responses, whereas chronic HP shifts to Th2 responses and is associated with lung fibrosis [20, 21]. CCL17, one of Th2 chemokines and also called TARC (Thymus and activation-regulated chemokines), and its receptor CCR4 induce lung fibrosis with alveolar macrophage migration in bleomycin-injured mice [22]. In bird-related HP, high serum CCL17/CXCL10 (Th1 chemokine) ratio and CCR4/CXCR3 (receptor for CXCL10, Th1 chemokine) expression ratio in surgical lung biopsy were associated with UIP pattern [20]. High serum CCL17 and low serum CXCL9 (IFN-γ-inducible Th1 chemokine) are associated with a decline in lung function, and serum CCL17 correlates with the severity of lung fibrosis on chest HRCT [23]. In addition, patients with elevated serum CCL17 at the time of diagnosis of chronic HP had a significantly higher incidence of acute exacerbations than those without elevation, suggesting that Th2 chemokines may be involved in the development of acute exacerbations [24].

Periostin, an extracellular matrix protein with a molecular weight of 90 kDa, is an inducible product of the Th2 cytokines IL-4 and IL-13. Serum periostin is a promising biomarker as a predictor of pulmonary fibrosis and worsening pulmonary function [25]. This biomarker also correlates with fibrosis score and poor prognosis of chronic HP, suggesting that it may be a biomarker for fibrosis and prognosis in HP [26].

Th1 and Th17 cytokines are important for the immune response in the acute phase of HP [27]. CXCL9, Th1 cytokine that binds with CXCR3, is a candidate for the biomarker of HP. CXCL9 expression and granuloma formation were attenuated with IFN-γ knockout in HP model mouse with *Saccharopolyspora rectivirgula* [28]. CXCL9 expression in the lung is upregulated in HP patients compared to IPF patients, and higher serum CXCL9 is also associated with the milder decline in lung function, suggesting that CXCL9 is not only a diagnostic biomarker for HP, but also may act protective in HP [23, 29].

4 Others (CA15–3, RAGE, Autoantibodies)

Carcinoma antigen 15–3 (CA15–3) and soluble receptor for advanced glycation end-products (sRAGE) are not only the candidate biomarkers for IPF, but also reflect the pathogenesis of HP. CA15–3 is derived from MUC1 and is widely measured as a tumor marker for many types of cancer, especially breast cancer. Elevated serum CA15–3 also reflects type II alveolar epithelial cell damage and is elevated in IPF and sarcoidosis with advanced lung lesions [30, 31]. Serum CA15–3 decreased after treatment in patients with HP, and the decline of CA15–3 was associated with a better prognosis [32]. sRAGE acts as a decoy to capture advanced glycation end-products (AGEs) and is involved in oxidative reactions. The serum AGE/sRAGE ratio was elevated in IPF and chronic HP compared to healthy subjects [33]. Autoantibodies such as antinuclear antibody were positive in 15% (18/120) of patients with chronic HP, and the presence of autoantibody was an independent poor prognostic factor for HP [34]. These biomarkers are not specific to HP but may be useful in clinical practice for diagnosis and prognostic evaluation. Future prospective studies at multiple centers are warranted, as the majority of these studies were small and studied retrospectively.

References

1. Kohno N, Awaya Y, Oyama T, et al. KL-6, a mucin-like glycoprotein, in bronchoalveolar lavage fluid from patients with interstitial lung disease. Am Rev Respir Dis. 1993;148:637–42.
2. Ohtsuki Y, Nakanishi N, Fujita J, et al. Immunohistochemical distribution of SP-D, compared with that of SP-A and KL-6, in interstitial pneumothe nias. Med Mol Morphol. 2007;40:163–7.
3. Takahashi T, Munakata M, Ohtsuka Y, et al. Serum KL-6 concentrations in dairy farmers. Chest. 2000;118:445–50.
4. Inase N, Ohtani Y, Usui Y, et al. Chronic summer-type hypersensitivity pneumonitis: clinical similarities to idiopathic pulmonary fibrosis. Sarcoidosis Vasc Diffuse Lung Dis. 2007;24:141–7.
5. Tsushima K, Fujimoto K, Yoshikawa S, et al. Hypersensitivity pneumonitis due to Bunashimeji mushrooms in the mushroom industry. Int Arch Allergy Immunol. 2005;137:241–8.
6. Tsushima K, Furuya S, Yoshikawa S, et al. Therapeutic effects for hypersensitivity pneumonitis induced by Japanese mushroom (Bunashimeji). Am J Ind Med. 2006;49:826–35.
7. Yoshikawa S, Tsushima K, Yasuo M, et al. Hypersensitivity pneumonitis caused by Penicillium citrinum, not Enoki spores. Am J Ind Med. 2007;50:1010–7.
8. Janssen R, Grutters JC, Sato H, et al. Analysis of KL-6 and SP-D as disease markers in bird fancier's lung. Sarcoidosis Vasc Diffuse Lung Dis. 2005;22:51–7.
9. Ji Y, Bourke SJ, Spears M, et al. Krebs von den Lungen-6 (KL-6) is a pathophysiological biomarker of early-stage acute hypersensitivity pneumonitis among pigeon fanciers. Clin Exp Allergy. 2020;50:1391–9.
10. Inase N, Ohtani Y, Sumi Y, et al. A clinical study of hypersensitivity pneumonitis presumably caused by feather duvets. Ann Allergy Asthma Immunol. 2006;96:98–104.
11. Okamoto T, Fujii M, Furusawa H, et al. The usefulness of KL-6 and SP-D for the diagnosis and management of chronic hypersensitivity pneumonitis. Respir Med. 2015;109:1576–81.
12. Ohnishi H, Miyamoto S, Kawase S, et al. Seasonal variation of serum KL-6 concentrations is greater in patients with hypersensitivity pneumonitis. BMC Pulm Med. 2014;14:129.
13. Okamoto T, Tsutsui T, Suhara K, et al. Seasonal variation of serum KL-6 and SP-D levels in bird-related hypersensitivity pneumonitis. Sarcoidosis Vasc Diffuse Lung Dis. 2015;31:364–7.
14. Tsutsui T, Miyazaki Y, Okamoto T, et al. Antigen avoidance tests for diagnosis of chronic hypersensitivity pneumonitis. Respir Investig. 2015;53:217–24.
15. Hanzawa S, Tateishi T, Ishizuka M, et al. Changes in serum KL-6 levels during short-term strict antigen avoidance are associated with the prognosis of patients with fibrotic hypersensitivity pneumonitis caused by avian antigens. Respir Investig. 2020;58:457–64.
16. Onishi Y, Kawamura T, Higashino T, et al. Clinical features of chronic summer-type hypersensitivity pneumonitis and proposition of diagnostic criteria. Respir Investig. 2020;58:59–67.
17. Mostafa AI, Ahmed HAM, Bayoumi AI, et al. Role of Krebs von den lungen-6 (KL-6) in assessing hypersensitivity pneumonitis. Tuberc Respir Dis (Seoul). 2021;84:200–8.
18. Ohnishi H, Yokoyama A, Yasuhara Y, et al. Circulating KL-6 levels in patients with drug induced pneumonitis. Thorax. 2003;58:872–5.
19. Ohnishi H, Yokoyama A, Hamada H, et al. Humidifier lung: possible contribution of endotoxin-induced lung injury. Intern Med. 2002;41:1179–82.
20. Kishi M, Miyazaki Y, Jinta T, et al. Pathogenesis of cBFL in common with IPF? Correlation of IP-10/TARC ratio with histological patterns. Thorax. 2008;63:810–6.
21. Inoue Y, Ishizuka M, Furusawa H, et al. Acute inflammatory and immunologic responses against antigen in chronic bird-related hypersensitivity pneumonitis. Allergol Int. 2019;68:321–8.
22. Belperio JA, Dy M, Murray L, et al. The role of the Th2 CC chemokine ligand CCL17 in pulmonary fibrosis. J Immunol. 2004;173:4692–8.
23. Nukui Y, Yamana T, Masuo M, et al. Serum CXCL9 and CCL17 as biomarkers of declining pulmonary function in chronic bird-related hypersensitivity pneumonitis. PLoS One. 2019;14:e0220462.

24. Miyazaki Y, Unoura K, Tateishi T, et al. Higher serum CCL17 may be a promising predictor of acute exacerbations in chronic hypersensitivity pneumonitis. Respir Res. 2013;14:57.
25. Okamoto M, Hoshino T, Kitasato Y, et al. Periostin, a matrix protein, is a novel biomarker for idiopathic interstitial pneumonias. Eur Respir J. 2011;37:1119–27.
26. Nukui Y, Miyazaki Y, Masuo M, et al. Periostin as a predictor of prognosis in chronic bird-related hypersensitivity pneumonitis. Allergol Int. 2019;68:363–9.
27. Ishizuka M, Miyazaki Y, Masuo M, et al. Interleukin-17A and neutrophils in a murine model of bird-related hypersensitivity pneumonitis. PLoS One. 2015;10:e0137978.
28. Nance S, Cross R, Fitzpatrick E. Chemokine production during hypersensitivity pneumonitis. Eur J Immunol. 2004;34:677–85.
29. Furusawa H, Cardwell JH, Okamoto T, et al. Chronic hypersensitivity pneumonitis, an interstitial lung disease with distinct molecular signatures. Am J Respir Crit Care Med. 2020;202:1430–44.
30. Ricci A, Mariotta S, Bronzetti E, et al. Serum CA 15-3 is increased in pulmonary fibrosis. Sarcoidosis Vasc Diffuse Lung Dis. 2009;26:54–63.
31. Moll SA, Wiertz IA, Vorselaars AD, et al. Serum biomarker CA 15-3 as predictor of response to antifibrotic treatment and survival in idiopathic pulmonary fibrosis. Biomark Med. 2020;14:997–1007.
32. Moll SA, Wiertz IA, Vorselaars AD, et al. Change in serum biomarker CA 15-3 as an early predictor of response to treatment and survival in hypersensitivity pneumonitis. Lung. 2020;198:385–93.
33. Machahua C, Montes-Worboys A, Planas-Cerezales L, et al. Serum AGE/RAGEs as potential biomarker in idiopathic pulmonary fibrosis. Respir Res. 2018;19:215.
34. Adegunsoye A, Oldham JM, Demchuk C, et al. Predictors of survival in coexistent hypersensitivity pneumonitis with autoimmune features. Respir Med. 2016;114:53–60.

Chapter 9
Pathology

How Does Pathology Contribute to the Diagnosis of HP?

Tamiko Takemura

1 Introduction

Hypersensitivity pneumonitis (HP) is an immunologically mediated interstitial lung disease caused by inhalation of various antigens in susceptible individuals [1]. The antigens are very numerous in the environment, and it is difficult to identify the exact causative antigens [2]. Higher incidence of HP has been recognized in various interstitial lung diseases [3, 4], but it has been difficult to differentiate between chronic HP and idiopathic pulmonary fibrosis (IPF) [5, 6]. Furthermore, the cases in which antigens could be detected revealed better prognosis than those without antigen detection comparable with that of IPF [7]. Thus, appropriate management of HP is needed. Two guidelines for diagnosis and management of HP have been published, in 2020 [8] and 2021 [9], respectively, and both guidelines classified HP into nonfibrotic and fibrotic HP instead of acute, subacute and chronic HP.

2 The Distribution of Inhaled Antigens in the Lungs

Inhaled particles, measuring less than 2.5 μm, are easily deposited at the respiratory bronchiole level through diffusion. They are then phagocytized by alveolar macrophages, and move to peripheral areas adjacent to the interlobular lymphatic vessels. An antigen inhalation experiment in mice revealed that the inhaled antigens were mostly deposited at the respiratory bronchiole and alveolar duct level [10]. The lymphatic vessels in the lung are composed of interstitial and venous systems and

T. Takemura (✉)
Department of Pathology, Kanagawa Cardiovascular and Respiratory Center, Yokohama, Japan

Y. Miyazaki (ed.), *Hypersensitivity Pneumonitis*, Respiratory Disease Series: Diagnostic Tools and Disease Managements,
https://doi.org/10.1007/978-981-96-7983-6_9

broncho-vascular bundles and ultimately drain into the pulmonary hilar region [11]. The lymphatic vessels in the lungs are more numerous in the upper zones than in the lower lobes [12].

3 Diagnostic Procedure for HP

In cases of nonfibrotic HP, which are usually in the acute phase of HP, the typical histological features can be easily detected by transbronchial lung biopsy (TBLB) specimens. The diagnostic findings of nonfibrotic HP mainly consist of lymphocytic bronchiolitis, cellular IP (like cellular NSIP), and poorly formed granulomas, and they can be detected by examination of TBLB specimens in 46% of HP cases in addition to. bronchoalveolar lavage [13].

While cellular HP can be accurately diagnosed by TBLB, it is difficult to differentiate fibrotic HP from other fibrotic lung diseases by TBLB. Transbronchial lung cryobiopsy (TBLC) has recently been used as a useful diagnostic tool for diffuse parenchymal lung diseases [14, 15]. The ATS guideline suggests performing TBLC in patients with nonfibrotic HP, depending on the availability of local expertise [8]. The Chest guideline states that performing TBLC in HP requires that the pathologist be experienced and proficient and that its pathological diagnosis be supported by multidisciplinary discussion (MDD), the same as in various interstitial lung diseases [9].

3.1 Histopathological Findings of TBLB Specimens in Nonfibrotic HP

Figure 9.1 shows diffuse lymphocyte infiltration in the alveolar walls, scattered intra-alveolar polypoid fibrosis (Masson bodies), and loose granuloma, measuring less than 150 μm in the alveolar lumina, in a patient with summer-type HP.

3.2 Histpathological Findings of TBLC Specimens in Nonfibrotic HP

A properly obtained specimen by TBLC is composed of acini [16], and shows an airway-centered distribution of inflammatory cells and fibrosis. Figure 9.2 shows lymphocyte infiltration in the wall of a respiratory bronchiole and alveolar duct walls, intra-alveolar macrophages, and a giant cell granuloma with a cholesterol cleft that are observed in a patient with summer-type HP.

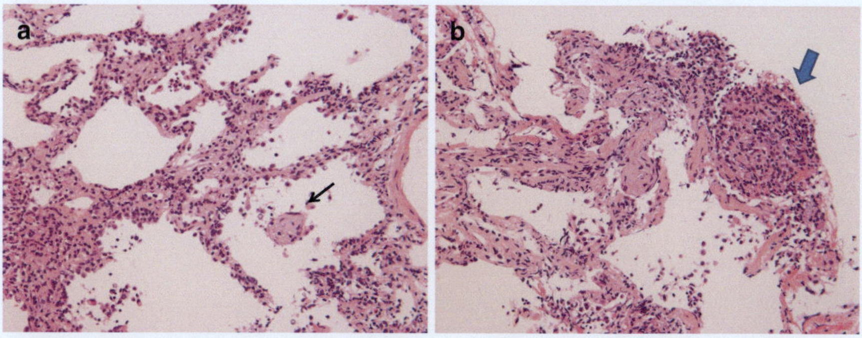

Fig. 9.1 Histological finding of transbronchial lung biopsy (TBLB) specimen of nonfibrotic HP of a patient with positive antibody to *Trichosporon asahi*. (**a**) Lymphocyte alveolitis and a small intra-alveolar polypoid fibrosis (HE, ×10). (**b**) A loose granuloma (arrow) in the alveolar lumen (HE, ×20)

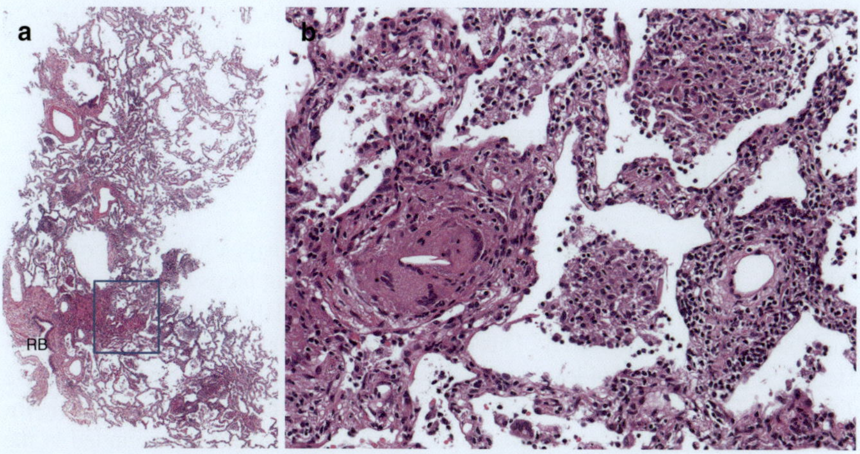

Fig. 9.2 Specimens taken from transbronchial lung cryobiopsy (TBLC). (**a** and **b**) Histology of nonfibrotic HP taken by TBLC of a patient with summer-type HP. (**a**) A panoramic view of TBLC specimen showing diffuse lymphocyte alveolitis and bronchiolitis (HE, ×2). (**b**) A giant cell granuloma with cholesterol cleft and lymphocyte alveolitis in a square of (**a**) (HE ×10). RB respiratory bronchiole

Figure 9.3 reveals a TBLC specimen of fibrotic HP, clearly demonstrating airway-centered fibrosis and a poorly formed granuloma in the wall of a respiratory bronchiole. However, it is not easy to differentiate between fibrotic HP and IPF/UIP or other fibrotic connective tissue diseases on the basis of the pathological findings in cryobiopsy specimens.

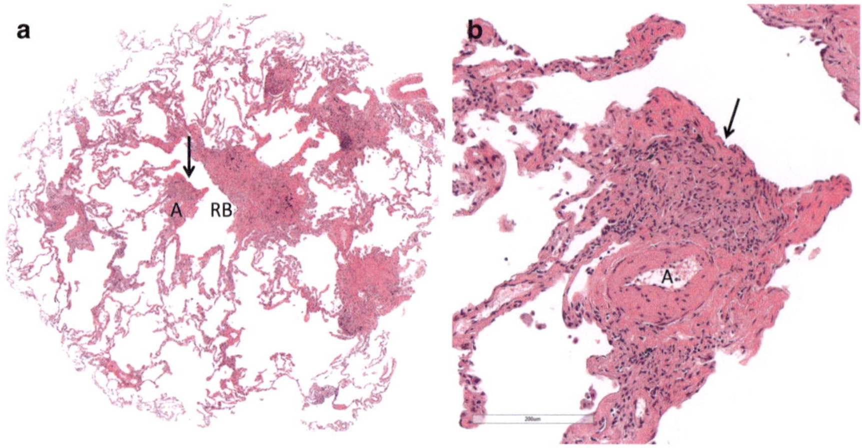

Fig. 9.3 Histology of fibrotic HP taken by TBLC. (**a**) A panoramic view of the specimen of fibrotic HP taken by TBLC. Patchy fibrosis, especially located at the centrilobular area (HE, ×2). RB, respiratory bronchiole. (**b**) A loose granuloma (arrow) in the wall of the respiratory bronchiole (HE, ×15). RB respiratory bronchiole, A pulmonary artery

4 Histopathology of Surgical Lung Biopsy Specimens in Nonfibrotic HP

Both the ATS and the Chest guidelines state that the histopathological criteria of nonfibrotic HP and fibrotic HP are based on surgical lung biopsy specimens [8, 9]. According to ATS guideline, nonfibrotic HP and fibrotic HP are classified as typical, probable, indeterminate for HP. This criterion may be based on IPF guideline [17]. The Chest guideline provides detailed descriptions of many diseases as alternative diagnoses. Thus it is indicated indeterminate for HP in the cases not applicable for typical or probable and alternative diagnosis. "Hot tub lung" was excluded in the criteria of nonfibrotic and /or fibrotic HP [8]. Table 9.1 shows histology of typical nonfibrotic HP, according to ATS and Chest guidelines.

4.1 Histopathology of Nonfibrotic HP

Basically, histological features of nonfibrotic HP are observed around the small airways, that is, airway-centered distribution. The histopathological findings in nonfibrotic HP consist of cellular bronchiolitis, predominant lymphocyte infiltration in the respiratory bronchiole to the alveolar duct, lymphocytic alveolitis (cellular NSIP pattern), and poorly formed granuloma (Figs. 9.4 and 9.5). The ATS and Chest guidelines both state that all three features of cellular IP, cellular bronchiolitis, and poorly formed granuloma are observed in at least one biopsy site in typical nonfibrotic HP. Intra-alveolar polypoid fibrosis (Masson body), and accumulation of foamy macrophage are sometimes seen in the alveolar lumina.

Table 9.1 Histopathological criteria for the diagnosis of typical nonfibrotic HP (ATS [8]/ Chest [9])

Nonfibrotic HP (ATS/JRS/ALAT 2020)	Typical nonfibrotic HP (Chest 2021)
At least one biopsy site showing all three of the following features 1. Cellular interstitial pneumonia Bronchiolocentric(airway-centered) Cellular NSIP pattern Lymphocyte-predominant 2. Cellular bronchiolitis Lymphocyte-predominant (Lymph > Plasma cells) with no more than focal peribronchiolar lymphoid aggregates with germinal centers ±Organizing pneumonia pattern with Masson bodies ±Foamy macrophages in terminal air spaces 3. Poorly formed non-necrotizing granulomas Loose clusters of epithelioid cells and/or multinucleated giant cells ± intracytoplasmic inclusions Situated in peribronchiolar interstitium, terminal air spaces, and/or organizing pneumonia (Masson bodies) and Absence of features in any biopsy site to suggest an alternative diagnosis Plasma cells > lymphocytes Extensive lymphoid hyperplasia Extensive well-formed sarcoidal granulomas and/or necrotizing granulomas Aspirated particulates	*Major features* Presence of all four major features in at least one of the sampled lobes of lung 1. Small airway distribution (bronchioles and/or alveolar ducts) 2. Uniform cellular interstitial inflammation of alveolar walls and bronchioles (cellular bronchiolitis); may include regions with a cellular NSIP pattern 3. Inflammation consisting of mostly lymphocytes 4. Interstitial scattered, usually single, poorly formed non-necrotizing granulomas and/or multinucleated giant cells *Minor features* (a) Organizing pneumonia, small foci (b) Foamy macrophages (c) Cholesterol clefts, Schaumann bodies, calcium oxalate crystals And Lack of features suggesting an alternative diagnosis

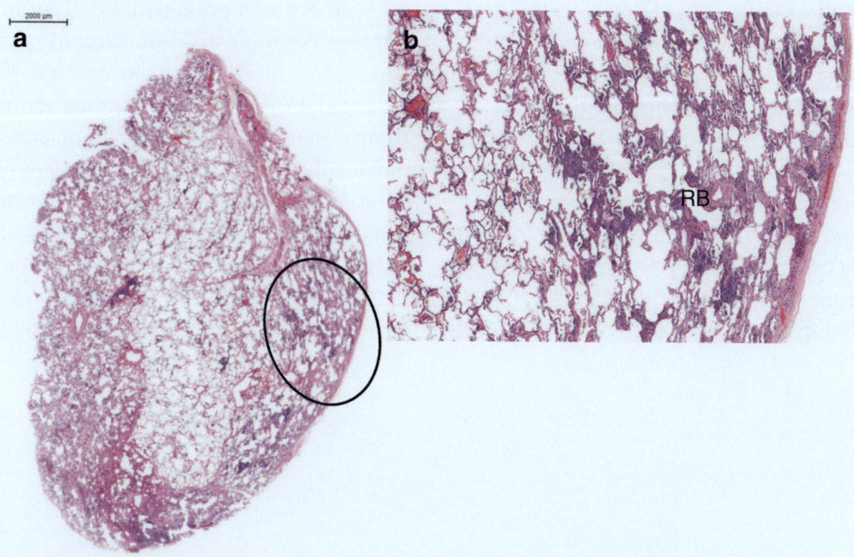

Fig. 9.4 Histology of nonfibrotic HP of surgical specimen. (**a**) A panoramic view of the right lower lobes shows diffuse lymphocyte alveolitis like cellular NSIP (HE, ×0.5). (**b**) Lymphocye-alveolitis prominently seen in the centriacinar area, indicated by a circle of (a). (HE, ×2) RB, respiratory bronchiole

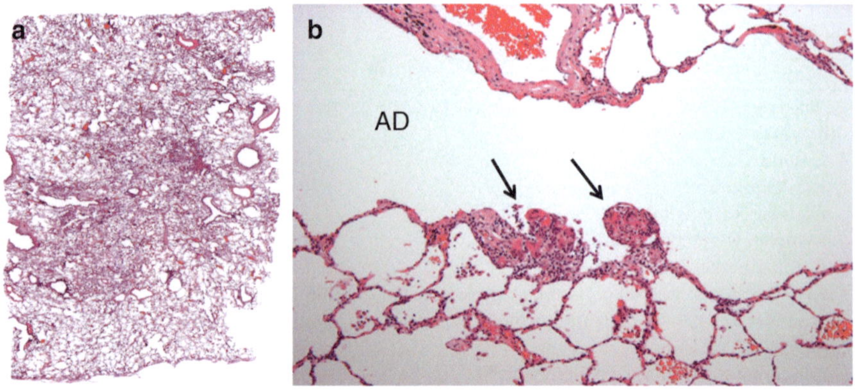

Fig. 9.5 Nonfibrotic HP of a bird-fancier. (**a**) Diffuse lymphocyte alveolitis, accentuated at the centrilobular area (HE, ×0.5) (**b**) Small poorly formed granulomas (arrows) are protruding to the alveolar duct (HE, ×20). AD, alveolar duct

In summer-type HP, lymphocytes infiltrating the alveolar walls are predominantly CD8 positive. Although lymphoid follicles are sometimes seen, marked lymphoid hyperplasia with germinal centers suggests an alternative diagnosis such as connective tissue disease.

The granulomas in nonfibrotic HP are observed in the bronchial and bronchiolar walls and also in the alveolar ducts and alveolar lumina. They are usually poorly formed nonnecrotizing granulomas smaller less than 150 μm, loose clusters of epithelioid cells, and/or multinucleated giant cells.

The giant cells occasionally contain intracytoplasmic inclusions, such as cholesterol clefts, Schaumann bodies (laminated calcifications), and asteroid bodies (Fig. 9.6). However, the presence of well-formed epithelioid cell granulomas with circumscribed hyalinized fibrosis is suggestive of sarcoidosis. The size and distribution of the granulomas seen in HP are summarized in Table 9.2. Minor histopathological features consist of small foci of organizing pneumonia (so-called Masson bodies), foamy macrophages, and giant cells with cholesterol clefts. Some cases of nonfibrotic HP resemble cases of pulmonary alveolar proteinosis showing PAS-positive proteinaceous material in the alveolar lumina (Fig. 9.7a). Occasionally, lymphocyte infiltration and accumulations of foamy macrophages in the alveolar lumina are seen, adjacent to the interlobular septum (Fig. 9.7b). Probable or compatible for Nonfibrotic HP reveals small airway distribution, cellular bronchiolitis, and

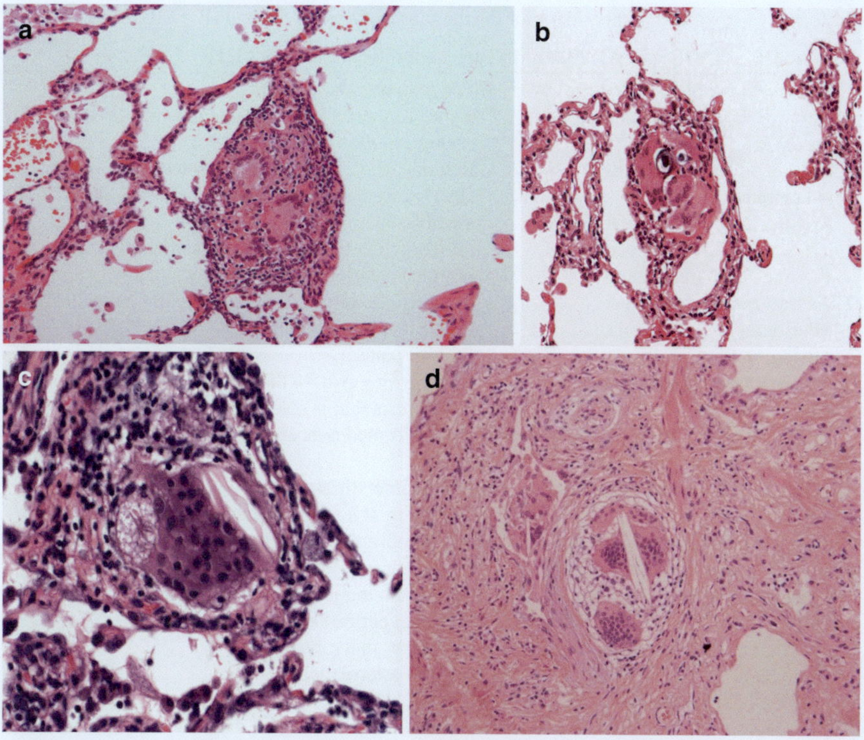

Fig. 9.6 Granulomas seen in nonfibrotic and fibrotic HP. (**a**) A granuloma consists of giant cells and lymphocytes in nonfibrotic HP (×20). (**b**) A granuloma consists of giant cells containing Schauman body (HE, ×20). (**c**) A giant cell has an asteroid body and cholesterol cleft with lymphocyte infiltration (HE, ×40). (**d**) Giant cell granuloma having cholesterol cleft is seen in the interstitium of fibrotic HP (HE, ×20)

lymphocyte predominant cellular IP except for poorly formed granuloma. Indeterminate for nonfibrotic HP does not meet criteria for nonfibrotic, probable (ATS) or typical, compatible, and alternative (Chest).

In Japan, ultrasonic room humidifiers are often used, especially during the winter season, and humidifer lung has been reported as a form of HP caused by inhalational exposure to the air disseminated by contaminated humidifiers [17]. Histology reveals the characteristic findings of nonfibrotic HP, that is, lymphocytic alveolitis, intra-alveolar polypoid fibrosis, and loose granuloma. Sometimes, PAS-positive proteinaceous materials like as alveolar proteinosis can be seen in cases of nonfibrotic HP (Fig. 9.7).

Table 9.2 Histopathological criteria for the diagnosis of typical fibrotic HP (ATS/Chest)

Fibrotic HP (ATS/JRS/ALAT 2020)	Typical fibrotic HP (Chest 2021)
Typical histopathological features of fibrotic HP, 1, 2,and 3 in at least one biopsy site: 1. Chronic fibrosing interstitial pneumonia Architectural distortion, fibroblast foci ± subpleural honeycombing Fibrotic NSIP-like pattern 2. Airway-centered fibrosis ±Peribronchiolar metaplasia ±Bridging fibrosis 3. Poorly formed non-necrotizing granulomas ±Cellular interstitial pneumonia ±Cellular bronchiolitis ±Organizing pneumonia pattern and Absence of features in any biopsy site to suggest an alternative diagnosis Plasma cells > lymphocytes Extensive well-formed sarcoid granulomas and/or necrotizing granulomas Aspirated particulates	*Major features* Presence of these two major features in at least one of the samples lobe 1. Regions where small airway-centered fibrosis is clearly present with or without peribronchiolar metaplasia 2. Fibrosing interstitial pneumonia affecting at least one sampled area/lobe of lung parenchyma with regions showing one or more of the following patterns (a) NSIP-fibrosing pattern (b) UIP pattern (c) Fibrosing pattern that is difficult to classify (d) Fibrosis that is solely peribronchiolar 3. Poorly formed noncaseating granulomas Or Fibrosing interstitial pneumonia meeting only major feature #2 in at least one lobe, as well as all criteria for typical nonfibrotic HP in a separate lobes *Minor features* (a) Organizing pneumonia, small foci. (b) Focal peribronchiolar metaplasia (c) Foamy macrophages (d) Cholesterol clefts *Lack of* Features of an alternative diagnosis

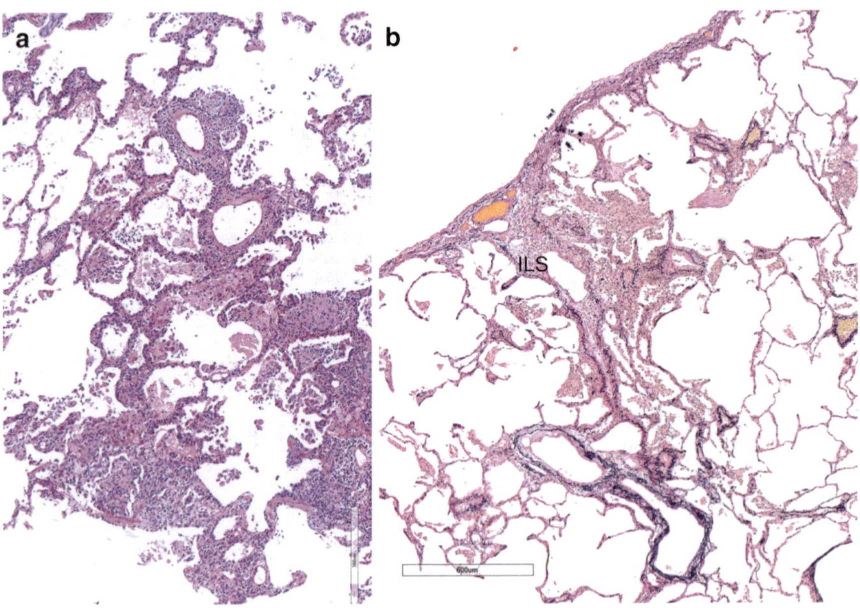

Fig. 9.7 (**a**) Intra-alveolar accumulation of PAS-positive proteinaceous exudates, and alveolar macrophage with lymphocyte alveolitis are seen in a summer-type HP (HE, ×10). (**b**) Lymphocyte and macrophage accumulate occasionally close to the interlobular septum (EVG, ×4) ILS, interlobular septum

5 Histopathology of Fibrotic HP

It is very difficult to make a diagnosis of fibrotic HP on the basis of the pathological findings, because it must be differentiated from numerous fibrotic interstitial pneumonias, including IPF and connective-tissue disease-associated interstitial pneumonia. The Chest guideline regarding the pathologic pattern of fibrotic HP may be comparable with the guideline regarding IPF [18]. Three major histologic features must be present in at least one of the lobes biopsied to make a pathological diagnosis of typical fibrotic HP [8, 9] (Table 9.3): (1) chronic fibrosing interstitial pneumonia with architectural distortion, fibroblastic foci, honeycombing, that is, a UIP pattern, or a fibrotic NSIP pattern, (2) airway-centered fibrosis with or without peribronchiolar metaplasia [19] and with or without bridging fibrosis [20], and (3) poorly formed noncaseating granulomas. Cellular interstitial pneumonia, cellular bronchiolitis, and organizing pneumonia can also be observed as minor features in fibrotic HP [8, 9]. Probable fibrotic HP is defined as two major features of chronic fibrosing IP (fibrosing NSIP pattern, UIP pattern, unclassifiable fibrosing pattern), and airway-centered fibrosis with or without bronchiolar metaplasia in at least one biopsy site, but no granuloma. Indeterminate for fibrotic HP, chronic fibrosing interstitial pneumonia can be at least one biopsy site. The Chest guideline describes fibrosing sarcoidosis, aspiration of fibrosis, fibrosing IP in connective tissue disease, and other diseases as alternative diagnoses. The ATS guideline describes several histological features whose presence suggests an alternative diagnosis, for example, that a predominance of plasma cells over lymphocytes suggests a diagnosis of connective-tissue-associated IP, and well-formed sarcoidal granulomas or necrotizing granuloma and aspirated particulates suggest alternative diseases.

High-resolution computed tomography (HRCT) shows ill-defined centrilobular nodules, mosaic attenuation, and three-density patterns of a bird-fancier (Fig. 9.8). Histology of surgical lung biopsy from the upper lobe shows subpleural and perilobular fibrosis, patchy airway-centered fibrosis, and peribronchiolar metaplasia. Poorly formed loose granulomas can be observed at a respiratory bronchiole (Fig. 9.9). The lower lobe of this case shows perilobular fibrosis with bridging fibrosis, corresponding to the HRCT image (Fig. 9.10). In the fibrotic HP, bridging fibrosis has often been observed between centrilobular region and the interlobular septum and/or subpleural region (Fig. 9.11). The most common pattern of bridging fibrosis consists of connection between the respiratory bronchiole and interlobular septum [20]; thus, the distance between respiratory bronchiole and interlobular septum becomes too short. Most cases showing hexaginal pattern on HRCT [21] are diagnosed as probable fibrotic HP [21] showing UIP and airway-centered fibrosis without granuloma. Probable fibrotic HP must be differentiated from other forms of fibrosing IP with airway-centered fibrosis [22, 23].

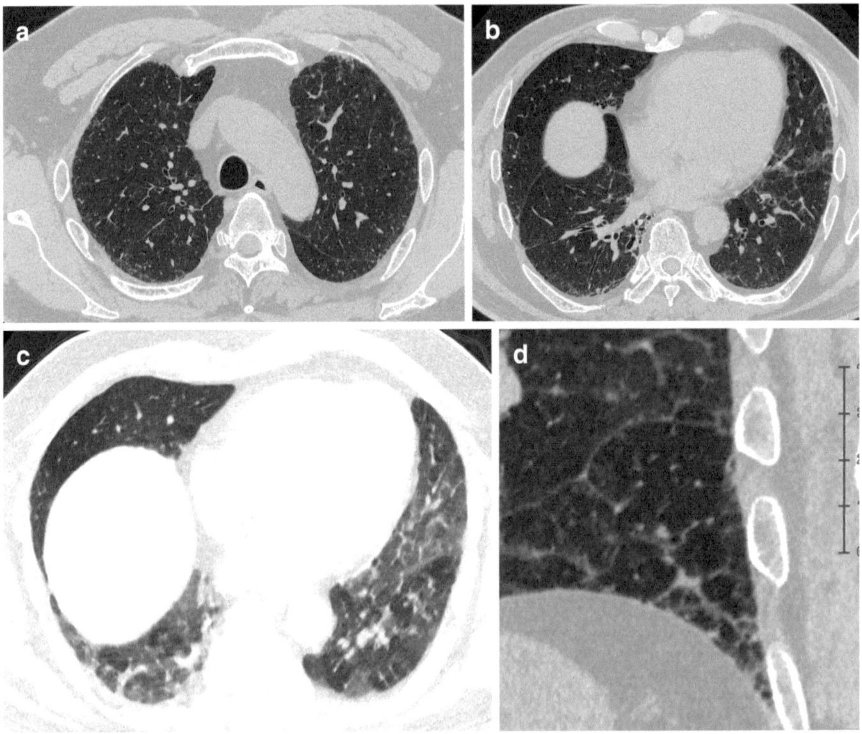

Fig. 9.8 HRCT scan images of a fibrotic HP of bird-fancier. (**a** and **b**) HRCT shows random distribution of ill-defined centrilobular nodular lesions, both axially and craniocaudally. (**c**) Air trapping on expiratory image. (**d**) A hexagonal pattern is seen in the lower lobe. (Courtesy of Dr. Tae Iwasawa, Department of Raidology, Kanagawa Cardiovascular and Respiratory Center)

6 Histologic Separation between Hypersentivity Pneumonia and Other Interstitial Lung Diseases

Poorer agreement in regard to the diagnosis of fibrotic HP in comparison with IPF and connective tissue diseases among experienced MDD groups has been reported [24]. Further antigen avoidance is recommended for the patients with HP. Although identification and avoidance of antigens are important for the management of HP patients, it is very difficult to identify the antigens [2, 6]. Further antigen avoidance is associated with improved survival in patients with chronic HP [7, 25].

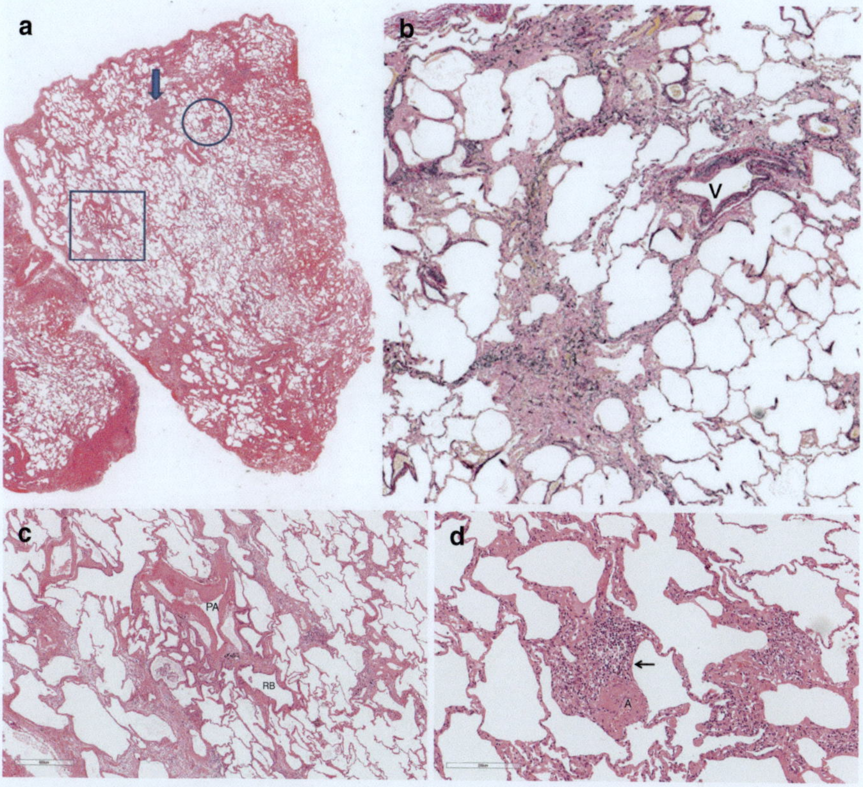

Fig. 9.9 Histology of typical fibrotic HP of a bird-fancier. (**a**) A specimen taken from left S1 + 2, showing subpleural fibrosis, perilobular fine fibrosis, and airway-centered fibrosis (arrow) (HE, ×0.5). (**b**) Airway-centered fibrosis (EVG, ×5) (arrow of a). V, vein. (**c**) A square shows pribronchiolar metaplasia (HE, ×4). RB respiratory bronchiole, PA Pulmonary artery. (**d**) A poorly formed granuloma (arrow) in the respiratory bronchiole wall (a circle of a). (HE, ×10) A, pulmonary artery

Fig. 9.10 The lower lobe of the case shown in Fig. 9.9. A panoramic view of S9 taken from the same case, showing subpleural and interlobular fibrosis and a centrilobular fibrosis (arrows), reflecting on hexagonal pattern on HRCT (Fig. 9.8d) (HE, ×0.5)

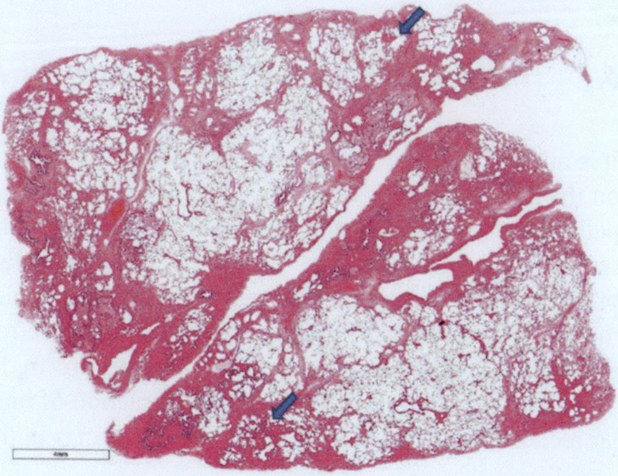

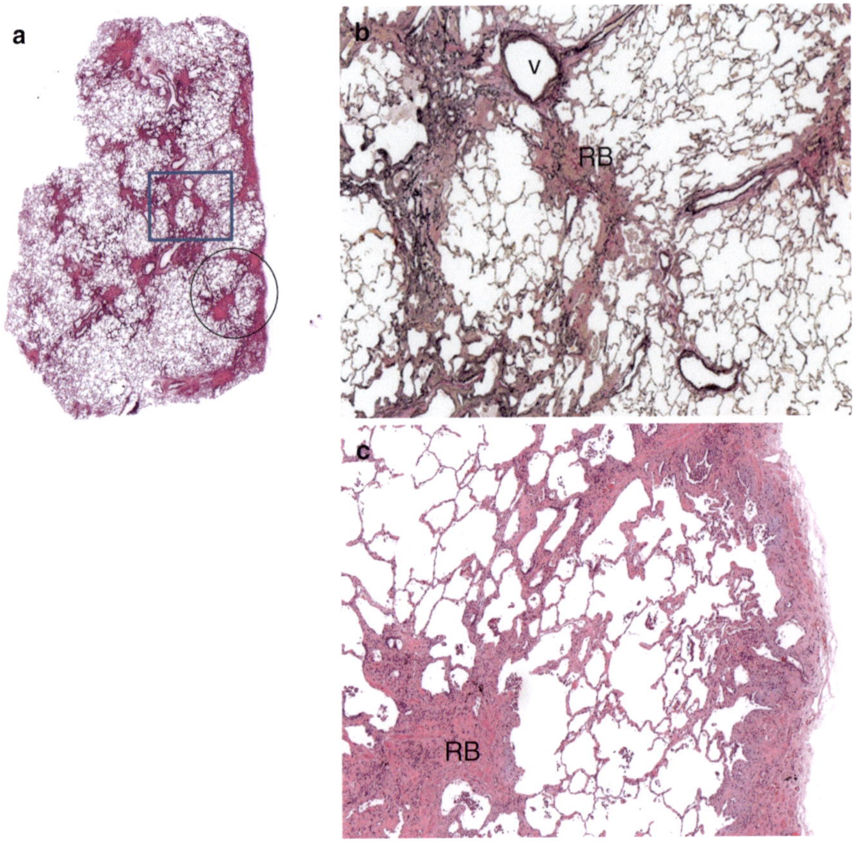

Fig. 9.11 Bridging fibrosis seen in a case of fibrotic HP of a bird-fancier. (**a**) A panoramic view of a specimen taken from the left lower lobe, showing subpleural and centrilobular fibrosis (arrow) (HE, ×0.5). V interlobular vein, RB respiratory bronchiole. (**b**) Centrilobular fibrosis is connecting to the interlobular and peiacinar interstitium in the square of **a** (EVG, ×4), corresponding to bridging fibrosis. (**c**) Dense centrilobular fibrosis (a circle of **a**) extends to the pleura (HE, ×4)

6.1 Histologic Differentiation from IPF/UIP

It is difficult to differentiate between fibrotic HP and progressive fibrosing IP based on the histopathological features, even if guidelines have been submitted. Several pathological features in fibrotic HP and IPF have been compared. Takemura et al. reported a higher frequency of bronchiolitis, centrilobular fibrosis, frequency of bridging fibrosis, organizing pneumonia, loose granuloma that are more prevalent than histological features of IPF [20]. Churg et al. reported a high frequency of peribronchiolar fibrosis and bridging fibrosis are frequent those in IPF/UIP [26]. Wright subsequently reported increased fraction of bronchioles with peribronchiolar metaplasia, presence of giant cells/granulomas in fibrotic HP than IPF/UIP, and no difference in the frequency of bridging fibrosis [27]. Yang also described absence of granulomas/interstitial giant cells, peribronchiolar metaplasia, less prominent airway centering, and prominent fibroblastic foci, which are key pathologic features of IPF/UIP in the differential diagnosis of HP from IPF/UIP [28].

Recently, Marinescu and experts reported the integration and application of the guidelines for IPF and fibrotic HP and emphasized multidisciplinary discussion [29].

6.2 Histological Differentiation from Connective Tissue Disease

It is usually difficult to differentiate between fibrotic HP and connective tissue disease (CTD) associated interstitial lung disease (ILD), because the histological features do often overlap. The guidelines suggest that a greater increase in plasma cell infiltration than lymphocyte infiltration, and the presence of extensive lymphoid hyperplasia positively favor connective diseases [8]. Churg compared the histologic features in12 cases of CTD-ILD and 16 cases of fibrotic HP [30], and reported finding that germinal centers, lymphoid aggregates, and plasma cells were more prominent in the lung in CTD-ILD cases, while peribronchiolar metaplasia fraction of bronchioles was more prominent in the lung in the cases of fibrotic HP.

7 Hypersensitivity Pneumonitis with Connective Tissue Diseases

It is well known that some HP patients have an autoimmune disease such as HPAF [31]. The patients, predominantly female, had a diagnosis of autoimmune disease such as scleroderma, Sjogren's disease, and so on.

Histological examination of lung specimens from HPAF cases have shown hyperplasia of lymphoid follicles and an increase in plasma cells in addition to histological characteristics of HP (Fig. 9.12).

8 Lung Transplantation for Fibrotic HP

Lung transplantation has recently been performed in cases of fibrotic HP with progressive fibrosis, and Kern et al. have reported longer survival times after transplantation, in comparison with IPF patients [32]. However, vigilance for antigen exposure and disease recurrence is important after lung transplantation for HP. Hanzawa reported a case of lung transplantation in a case of chronic bird fancier's lung [33], and surgical specimen revealed centrilobular, subpleural,

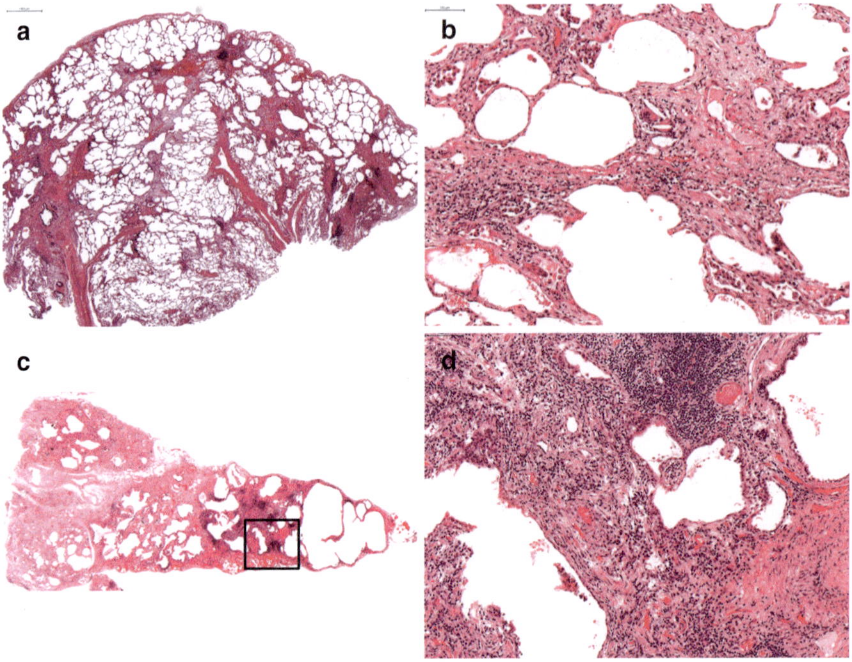

Fig. 9.12 A case of fibrotic HP developed to rheumatoid arthritis 9 year later. (**a**) A surgical lung biopsy from left S1 + 2 shows each connecting centrilobular and perilobular fibrosis (HE, ×1). (**b**) Aggregate of giant cells with cholesterol cleft is present in the fibrotic area (HE, ×10). (**c**) The lower lobe of this case shows cystic lesion with inflammatory cell infiltration (HE, ×1). (**d**) Prominent infiltration of plasma cells and a lymphoid follicle are seen in the fibrotic area indicated by square of Fig. 9.12 c(HE, ×20)

and perilobular fibrosis with bridging fibrosis, and a poorly formed granuloma as shown in Fig. 9.9. Eight years after the diagnosis, the patient's pulmonary function worsened, and the lung transplantation was performed. The explanted left lung revealed more marked progressive centrilobular fibrosis and subpleural fibrosis than fibrosis of surgical lung biopsy (Fig. 9.13).

9 Autopsy Cases of Fibrotic HP

In 2009, Akashi and Takemura reported the histopathological features of 16 autopsy cases of chronic HP in comparison of 11 autopsy cases of IPF [34]. Nine of 16 cases of fibrotic HP showing predominant UIP were compared with 11 cases with IPF autopsy cases. The results showed that upper lobe dominant fibrosis, centrilobular

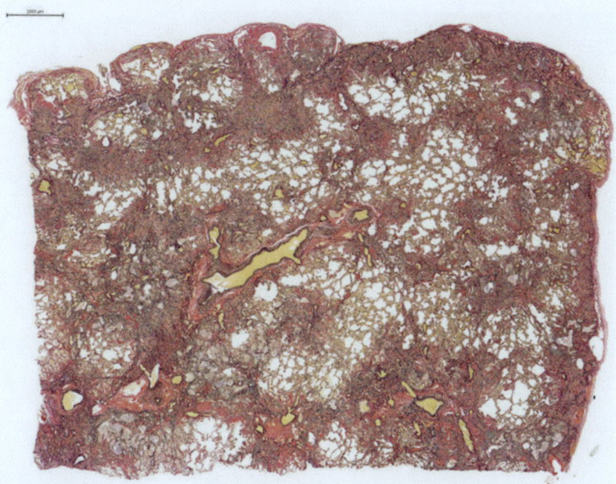

Fig. 9.13 A explanted left lung of a patient seen in Fig. 9.11. Compare with the histology of Fig. 9.11. A panoramic view of the lingula showing subpelural, perilobular, and prominent centrilobular dense fibrosis (EVG, ×0.5)

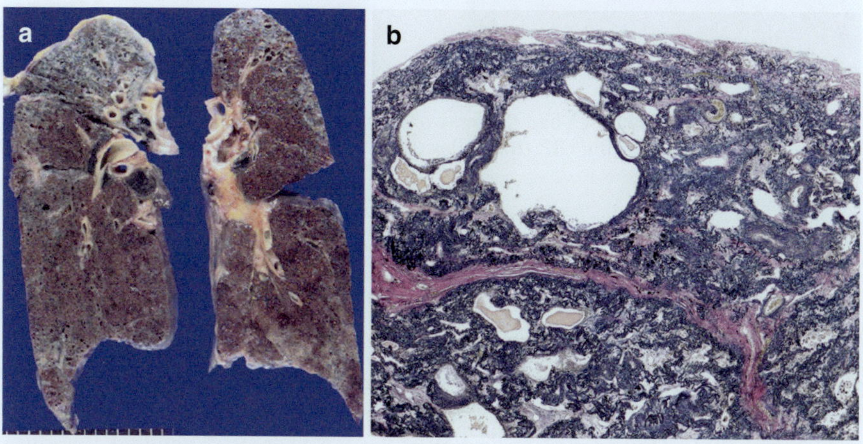

Fig. 9.14 (**a**) Autopsy lungs of a bird-fancier exposed by a large amount of bird extracts showing marked upper lobe contraction are noted. (**b**) The panoramic view shows marked atelectasis with elastosis of the upper lobe (EVG, ×1)

fibrosis, and bridging fibrosis were more common histological findings in the chronic HP cases than in the IPF cases. In the cases of upper lobe contraction, fibroelastosis was often observed (Fig. 9.14). There was no significant difference between chronic HP and IPF/UIP in the frequency of honeycomb lesions in the lower lobe (Fig. 9.15). The bridging fibrosis between centrilobular area and perilobular area was an outstanding feature. All nine of the 16 autopsy cases exhibited diffuse alveolar damage, same as in the IPF/UIP cases.

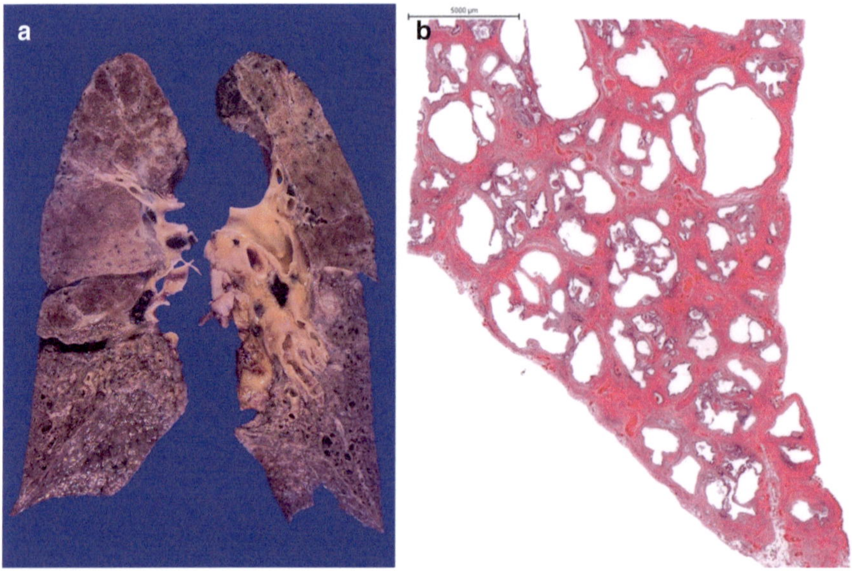

Fig. 9.15 (**a**) Autopsy lungs of a bird fancier, with a small amount bird extract in the long duration, are similar to those of IPF/UIP. (**b**) The lower lobe shows honeycombing, similar to that of IPF (HE, ×1) (**c**)

10 Conclusion

Because it is crucial to differentiate between IPF and fibrotic HP, and both diseases entail progressive fibrosis, HP guidelines were proposed by the ATS in 2020 and by the Chest in 2021. However, identification of the exact causative antigens continues to be difficult. Multidisciplinary discussion among the respirologists, radiologists, and pathologists is important to make the final diagnosis and decide on the management of fibrotic HP.

References

1. Costabel U, Miyazaki Y, Pardo A, et al. Hypersensitivity pnuemonitis. Nat Rev Dis Primers. 2020;6(1):15.
2. Morisset J, Johannson KA, Jones KD, et al. Identification of diagnostic criteria for chronic hypersensitivity pneumonitis. An international modified Delphi survey. Am J Respir Crit Care Med. 2018;197:1038–44.
3. Lederer DJ, Martinez FJ. Idiopathic pulmonary fibrosis. N Engl J Med. 2018;378:1811–23.
4. Wijsenbeek M, Cottin V. Spectrum of fibrotic lung diseases. N Engl J Med. 2020;383:958–68.

5. Travis WD, et al. An official American Thoracic Society/European Respiratory Society Statement: update of the international multidisciplinary classification of the idiopathic interstitial pneumonias. Am J Respir Crit Care Med. 2013;188:733–48.
6. Morell F, Villar A, Montero MA, et al. Chronic hypersensitivity pneumonitis in patients diagnosed with idiopathic pulmonary fibrosis: a prospective case-cohort study. Lancet Respir Med. 2013;1:685–94.
7. Fernández Pérez ER, Swigris JJ, Forsson AV, et al. Identifying antigen is associated with improved survival in patients with chronic hypersensitivity pneumonitis. Chest. 2013;144:1644–51.
8. Raghu G, Remy-Jardin M, Ryerson CJ, et al. Diagnosis of hypersensitivity pneumonitis in adults. An official ATS/JRS/ALAT clinical practice guideline. Am J Respir Crit Care Med. 2020;202:e36–69.
9. Fernandez Perez ER, Travis WD, Lynch DA, et al. Diagnosis and evaluation of hypersensitivity pneumonitis: chest guidelines and expert panel reports-executive summary. Chest. 2021;160:e97–e156.
10. Mitaka K, Miyazaki Y, Yasui M, et al. Th2-biased immune responses are important in a murine model of chronic hypersensitivity pneumonitis. Int Arch Allergy Immunol. 2011;154:264–74.
11. Egashira R, Tanaka T, Imaizumi T, et al. Differential distribution of lymphatic clearance between upper and lower regions of the lung. Respirol. 2013;18:348–53.
12. Okada Y. Pulmonary lymphatic system and lung cancer. 1st ed. Shiga: Kinpodo; 1989.
13. Adams TN, Newton CA, Batra K, et al. Utility of bron choalveolar lavage and transbronchial biopsy in patients with hypersensitivity pneumonitis. Lung. 2018;196(5):617–22.
14. Ravaglia C, Wells AU, Tomassetti A, et al. Diagnostic yield and risk/benefit analysis of transbronchial lung cryobiopsy in diffuse parenchymal lung disease: a large cohort of 699 patients. Pulm Med. 2019;19:16.
15. Hetzel J, Maldonado F, Ravaglia C, et al. Transbronchial cryobiopsies for the diagnosis of diffuse parenchymal lung diseases: expert statement from the cryobiopsy working group on safety and utility and a call for standardization of the procedure. Respiration. 2018;95:188–200.
16. Takemura T, Baba T, Niwa T, et al. Histology for transbronchial lung cryobiopsy samples. In: Poletti V, editor. Transbronchial cryobiopsy in diffuse parenchymal lung disease. Springer; 2019. p. 67–73.
17. Sakamoto S, Furukawa M, Shimizu H, et al. Clnical and radiological characteristics of ultrasonic humidifier lung and summer-type hypersensitivity pneumonitis. Res Med. 2020;174:106196.
18. Raghu G, Remy-Jardin M, Myers GL, et al. An official ATS/ERS/JRS/ALAT clinical practice guideline: diagnosis of idiopathic pulmonary fibrosis. Am J Respir Crit Care Med. 2018;198:e44–68.
19. Fukuoka J, Franks TJ, Colby TV, et al. Peribronchiolar metaplasia: a common histologic lesion in diffuse lung disease and a rare cause of interstitial lung disease: clinicopathologic features of 15 cases. Am J Surg Pathol. 2005;29:948–54.
20. Takemura T, Akashi T, Kamiya H, et al. Pathological differentiation of chronic hypersensitivity pneumonitis from idiopathic pulmonary fibrosis/usual interstitial pneumonia. Histopathology. 2012;61:1026–35.
21. Okabayashi H, Fukuda D, Iwasawa T, et al. The new useful high-resolution computed tomography finding for diagnosing fibrotic hypersensitivity penumonitis: "hexagonal pattern": a single-center retrospective study. BMC Pulm Med. 2022;22:76.
22. Kuranishi LT, Leslie KO, Ferreira RG, et al. Airway-centered interstitial fibrosis: etiology, clinical findings and prognosis. Respir Res. 2015;16:55.
23. Tanizawa K, Ley B, Vittinghoff E, et al. Significance of bronchiolocentric fibrosis in patients with histopathological usual interstitial pneumonia. Histopathology. 2019;74:1088–97.
24. Walsh SLF, Wells AU, Desai SR, et al. Multcentre evaluation of multidisciplinary team meeting agreement on diagnosis in diffuse parenchymal lung disease: a case-cohort study. Lancer Respir Med. 2016;4:557–65.

25. Petnak T, Thongprayoon BM, Ryu JH, Moua T. Antigen identification and avoidance on outcomes in fibrotic hypersensitivity pneumonitis. Eur Respir J. 2022;60:2101336.
26. Churg A, Bilawick A, wright JL. Pathology of chronic hypersensitivity pneumonitis. What is it? What are the diagnostic criteria? Why do we care? Arch Pathol Lab Med. 2018;142(1):109–19.
27. Wright JL, Churg A, Hague CJ, et al. Pathologic separation of idiopathic pulmonary fibrosis from fibrotic hypersensitivity pneumonitis. Mod Pathol. 2020;33:616–25.
28. Yang S-R, Beasley MB, Churg A, et al. Diagnosis of hypersensitivity pneumonitis. Review and summary of American College of Chest Physicians statement. Am J Surg Pathol. 2022;46:e71–93.
29. Marinescu D-C, Raghu G, Remy-Jardin M, et al. Integration and application of clinical practice guidelines for the diagnosis of idiopathic pulmonary fibrosis and fibrotic hypersensitivity pneumonitis. Chest. 2022;162:614–29.
30. Churg A, Wright JL, Ryerson CJ. Pathologic separation of chronic hypersensitivity pneumonitis from fibrotic connective tissue disease-associated interstitial lung disease. Am J Surg Pathol. 2017;41:1403–9.
31. Adegunsoye A, Oldham JM, Demchuk C, et al. Predictors of survival in coexistent hypersensitivity pneumonitis with autoimmune features. Res Med. 2016;114:53–60.
32. Kern RM, Singer JP, Koth L, et al. Lung transplantation for hypersensitivity pneumonitis. Chest. 2015;147:1558–65.
33. Hanzawa S, Tateishi T, Takemura T, et al. The analysis of surgical lung biopsy and explanted lung specimens shed light on the pathological progression of chronic bird-related hypersensitivity pneumonitis. Intern Med. 2019;58:1145–50.
34. Akashi T, Takemura T, Ando N, et al. Histopathologic analysis of sixteen autopsy cases of chronic hypersensitivity pneumonitis and comparison with idiopathic pulmonary fibrosis/usual interstitial pneumonia. Am J Clin Pathol. 2009;131:405–15.

Chapter 10
HRCT

How Does HRCT Contribute to Diagnosis of HP?

Takeshi Johkoh

1 Clinical Question

How does HRCT contribute to diagnosis of HP?

- Although HRCT findings of HP are nonspecific, CT diagnostic criteria, which are an admixture of such findings, contribute to multidisciplinary diagnosis (MDD) of HP.

2 General HRCT Findings in HP

2.1 Nonfibrotic HP (Mainly Previous Acute and Subacute HP)

HRCT findings consist of areas of ground-glass opacity and ill-defined, small centrilobular faint opacities on inspiratory scans (Fig. 10.1). These findings are diffusely distributed in the bilateral lung fields [1, 2]. Mosaic or three-density patterns (Fig. 10.1), which means admixture of high or low attenuated lobules and normal ones, are sometimes seen [2]. Distribution is predominantly diffuse in the craniocaudal direction, and the basal lung zones are often relatively spared [3].

T. Johkoh (✉)
Department of Radiology, Kansai Rosai Hospital, Amagaski, Japan

Y. Miyazaki (ed.), *Hypersensitivity Pneumonitis*, Respiratory Disease Series: Diagnostic Tools and Disease Managements,
https://doi.org/10.1007/978-981-96-7983-6_10

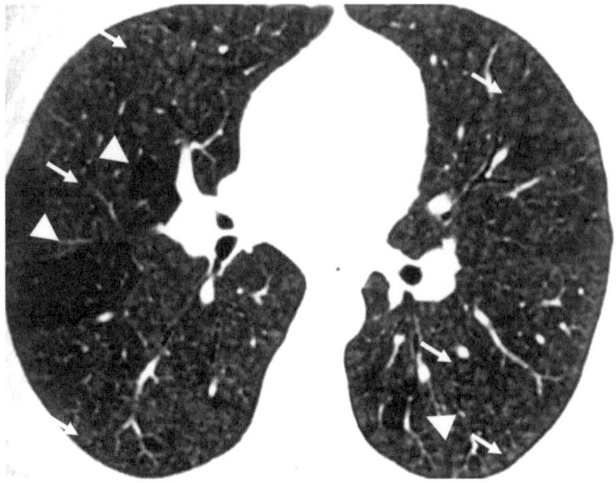

Fig. 10.1 HRCT of a 35-years-old male with nonfibrotic hypersensitivity pneumonitis. Centrilobular faint opacities superimposed (arrows) on areas of ground-glass opacities are diffusely distributed on HRCT. Low attenuated lobules are also seen (arrow heads)

2.2 *Fibrotic HP (Previously Called Chronic HP)*

Fibrotic HP, which has been previously described as chronic HP, is categorized into either recurrent or insidious types. Areas of ground-glass opacities are common in the recurrent type, which are accompanied by fibrotic findings such as honeycomb and traction bronchiectasis/bronchiectasis [4]. In the early stages, almost half of the lung field is occupied by ground-glass opacities, centrilobular nodules, and minimal fibrotic lesions. The proportion of ground-glass and nodular opacities is gradually decreasing. Almost 60% of the cases have fibrotic lesions that are distributed diffusely or mainly in the upper lung field; however, remaining approximately 40% of the cases have prominent fibrotic lesions in the lower field [5, 6]. A three-density pattern [7], which means an admixture of high or low attenuated lobules and normal ones, is commonly seen. Typically, ground-glass opacities are slightly less common in the insidious type compared to the recurrent one, and identifying distinct centrilobular nodular opacities is sometimes difficult. In many cases, differentiation from IPF is not easy owing to the accompanying honeycomb lung and severe traction bronchiectasis. In roughly estimated 20% of the cases, the prominent centrilobular opacities and the relatively random distribution of fibrotic findings in the craniocaudal direction made the diagnosis of fibrotic HP more easier when compared to that of IPF [8]. In addition, the subpleural compact consolidation with dilated air bronchiologram, called as pleuroparenchymal fibroelastosis, is sometimes seen in the upper lobe. In addition, a three-density pattern can also be observed in the insidious type.

3 HRCT Findings and Diagnosis According to the ATS/JRS/ALAT Guidelines

- Due to above-mentioned CT findings, the following CT diagnostic criteria are introduced [7]:

3.1 Nonfibrotic HP

3.1.1 Typical Nonfibrotic HP (Fig. 10.1)

Areas of ground-glass opacities or mosaic attenuation characterized by a patch work pattern of ground-glass opacities in combination with normal attenuation areas with diffuse craniocaudal and horizontal distribution are seen. These findings are suggestive of bronchiolar lesions that include ill-defined centrilobular nodules on the inspiratory scan and air trapping on the expiratory scan.

3.1.2 Compatible with Nonfibrotic HP (Fig. 10.2)

CT findings of nonfibrotic HP, which may not be typical but sometimes seen, are included. These include homogeneous areas of ground-glass opacities or airspace consolidations, and scattered thin-walled cysts. Lower and peribronchovascular predominance are also included.

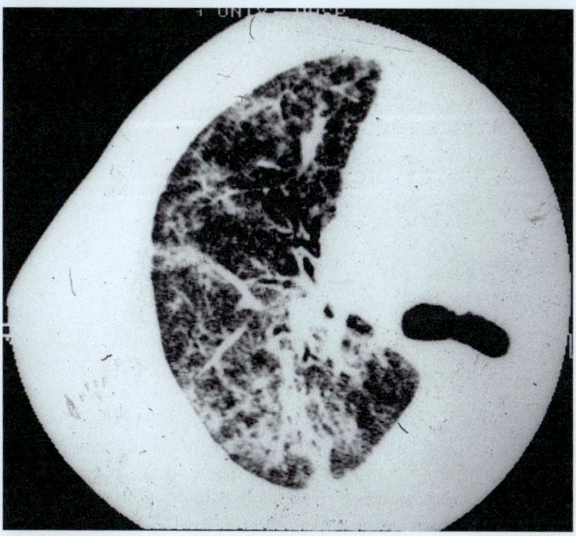

Fig. 10.2 HRCT of a 60-years-old male with nonfibrotic hypersensitivity pneumonitis. HRCT shows the admixture of areas of airspace consolidation and ground-glass opacities

3.2 *Fibrotic HP*

3.2.1 Typical Fibrotic HP (Fig. 10.3)

Typical fibrotic HP shows both fibrotic and bronchiolar ones, which show diffuse or random distribution in both craniocaudal and horizontal directions. This also includes cases with middle lung predominance as well as those with relative basal sparing.

3.2.2 Compatible with Fibrotic HP (Fig. 10.4)

Compatible with fibrotic HP is defined as coexisting fibrotic and bronchiolar lesions, with an uneven distribution of fibrotic lesions, such as upper or basal predominance craniocaudally, or peribronchovascular or central predominance. Cases with extensive areas of ground-glass opacities and minimal fibrosis are also included.

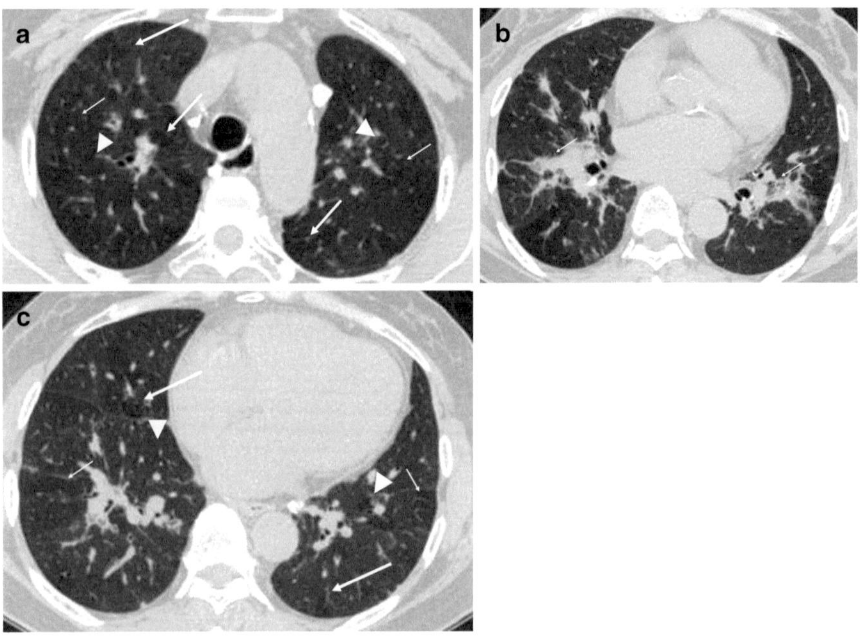

Fig. 10.3 HRCT of a 45-years-old male with fibrotic hypersensitivity pneumonia. (**a**) Low attenuated lobules (long arrows) are seen. Three-density pattern, which means admixture of low (long arrows) and high (arrows) attenuated lobules and normal lungs, is clearly seen. (**b**) In the middle lung zone, area of airspace consolidation with traction bronchiectasis (arrows) is quite prominent. (**c**) Low attenuated lobules (long arrows) are seen. Three-density pattern, which means admixture of low (long arrows) and high (arrows) attenuated lobules and normal lungs, is clearly seen. In this case, middle lung zone predominance is seen. Thus, this case is a typical fibrotic HP

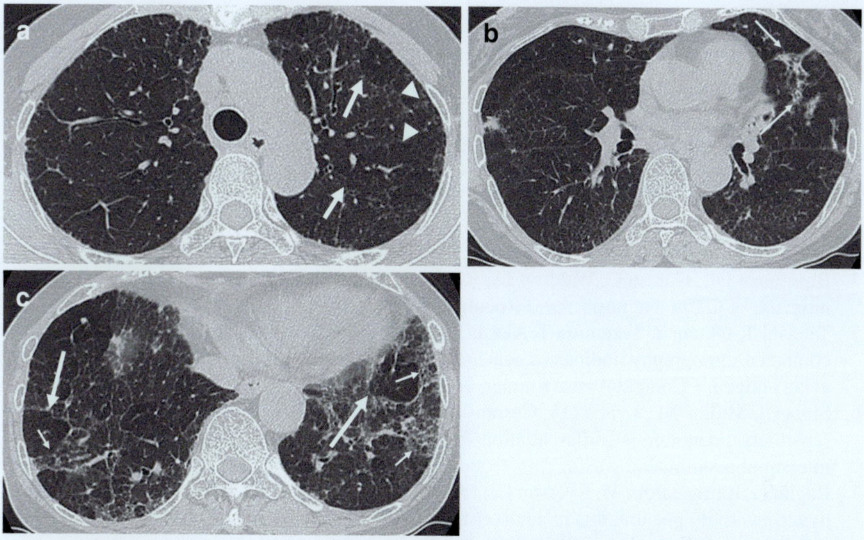

Fig. 10.4 HRCT of a 67-years-old male with fibrotic hypersensitivity pneumonitis. (**a**) Low attenuated lobules (arrows) and centrilobular nodules (arrow heads), which mean small airway diseases, are seen. (**b**) Areas with airspace consolidation having traction bronchiectasis (arrows) are found. (**c**) Low attenuated lobules (long arrows) are seen. Reticular opacities with traction bronchioloectasis (arrows) are distributed diffusely. This case shows lower lobe predominance. Thus, this is classified as compatible with fibrotic HP on CT

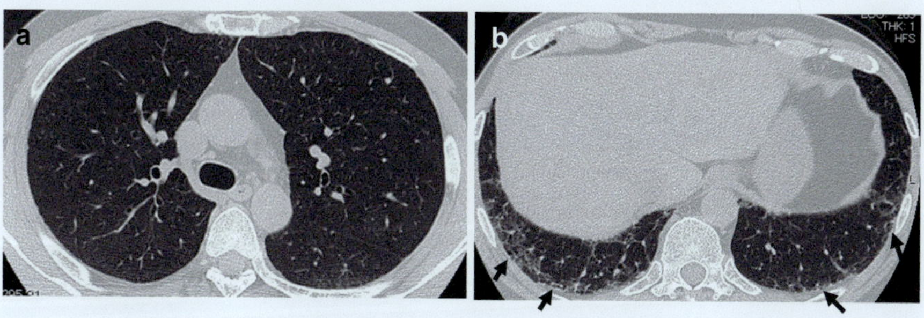

Fig. 10.5 HRCT of a 47-years-old male with fibrotic hypersensitivity pneumonitis. (**a** and **b**) In the basal subpleural lung fields, just reticular opacities with traction bronchioloectasis are seen (arrows). Thus, this case is classified as indeterminate for fibrotic HP

3.2.3 Indeterminate for Fibrotic HP (Fig. 10.5)

All the remaining cases of chronic fibrosing interstitial pneumonia are considered indeterminate for fibrotic HP. It is challenging to definitively classify these cases as fibrotic HP based solely on the imaging findings, especially when there are no strongly suggestive findings.

References

1. Lynch DA, Rose CS, Way D, King TE. Hypersensitivity pneumonitis: sensitivity of high-resolution CT in a population-based study. Am J Roentgenol. 1992;159:469–72.
2. Nakata H, Egashira K, Tsuda T, Hiraoka K, Kido M. High-resolution computed tomography of Japanese summer-type hypersensitivity pneumonitis. Clin Imag. 1991;15:185–90.
3. Rival G, Manzoni P, Lacasse Y, Polio JC, Westeel V, Dubiez A, et al. High- resolution CT predictors of hypersensitivity pneumonitis. Sarcoidosis, vasculitis, and diffuse lung diseases. Sarcoidosis Vasc Diffuse Lung Dis. 2016;33:117–23.
4. Buschman DL, Gamsu G, Waldron JA, Klein JS, King TE. Chronic hypersensitivity pneumonitis: use of CT in diagnosis. Am J Roentgenol. 1992;159:957–60.
5. Tateishi T, Ohtani Y, Takemura T, Akashi T, Miyazaki Y, Inase N, et al. Serial high-resolution computed tomography findings of acute and chronic hypersensitivity pneumonitis induced by avian antigen. J Comput Assist Tomogr. 2011;35:272–9.
6. Silva CI, Muller NL, Lynch DA, Curran-Everett D, Brown KK, Lee KS, et al. Chronic hypersensitivity pneumonitis: differentiation from idiopathic pulmonary fibrosis and nonspecific interstitial pneumonia by using thin-section CT. Radiology. 2008;246:288–97.
7. Raghu G, Remy-Jardin M, Ryerson CJ, Myers JL, Kreuter M, Vasakova M, et al. Diagnosis of hypersensitivity pneumonitis in adults. An official ATS/JRS/ALAT clinical practice guideline. Am J Respir Crit Care Med. 2020;202:e36–69.
8. Tateishi T, Johkoh T, Sakai F, Miyazaki Y, Ogura T, Ichikado K, et al. High- resolution CT features distinguishing usual interstitial pneumonia pattern in chronic hypersensitivity pneumonitis from those with idiopathic pulmonary f ibrosis. Jpn J Radiol. 2020;38:524–32.

Part III
Management and Prognosis

Chapter 11
Antigen Avoidance

How Much Does Antigen Avoidance Contribute to Treatments and Prognosis?

Yuki Iijima and Yasunari Miyazaki

1 Antigen Avoidance Test (AAT)

Antigen avoidance test (AAT) is a procedure to confirm a hallmark feature of hypersensitivity pneumonitis (HP) that elimination of the causative antigen leads to improvement of the disease. Especially in cases of nonfibrotic HP, patients often dramatically improve with the cessation of the culprit exposure alone. Therefore, spontaneous recovery after hospitalization strongly supports the diagnosis [1]. However, evaluating the diagnostic performance of the AAT for fibrotic HP is more challenging than for nonfibrotic HP. This is because fibrotic HP often progresses with long-term exposure to small amounts of antigen, making the impact of short-term antigen avoidance on the clinical course smaller. Indeed, very few reports have examined the significance of AATs for diagnosing or prognosis prediction of fibrotic HP. Tsutsui et al. studied 265 patients with suspected chronic HP who conducted AAT. The result revealed that just a 2-week antigen avoidance leading to an improvement in more than 2 out of 3 parameters, including vital capacity, Klebs von den Lungen-6 (KL-6), and white blood cell count (WBC), has a diagnostic value with a high specificity of 80.7%, while the sensitivity was low at 51.0% [2]. Okuda et al. also reported the utility of AAT for 40 patients with stable fibrotic HP [3]. As a result, an improvement in more than 2 out of 4 parameters, including KL-6, WBC or C-related protein, forced vital capacity, and imaging after 2-week antigen

Y. Iijima (✉)
Department of Respiratory Medicine, Institute of Science Tokyo, Tokyo, Japan
e-mail: iizima.pulm@tmd.ac.jp

Y. Miyazaki
Department of Respiratory Medicine, Tokyo Medical and Dental University, Bunkyo-ku, Tokyo, Japan
e-mail: miyazaki.pilm@tmd.ac.jp

Y. Miyazaki (ed.), *Hypersensitivity Pneumonitis*, Respiratory Disease Series: Diagnostic Tools and Disease Managements,
https://doi.org/10.1007/978-981-96-7983-6_11

avoidance was associated with a less decline in lung function, and a lower risk of death or acute exacerbation. However, both of these studies were retrospective studies at a single center, indicating limited evidence for the AAT, needing future prospective studies. The CHEST guideline also states that improvement with antigen avoidance supports the diagnosis of HP, but improvement may be ambiguous in several situations where the causative antigen is incorrect, antigen avoidance is incomplete, or fibrosis is highly advanced [4]. Therefore, while AAT is theoretically meaningful given the pathophysiology of HP, the evidence in actual clinical practice is lacking, requiring further evidence accumulation in the future.

2 Antigen Avoidance as a Treatment

Not only as a diagnostic value, but antigen avoidance is also a mainstay of the treatment. As mentioned above, many cases of nonfibrotic HP markedly improve with antigen avoidance alone, which also has an impact on the prognosis of fibrotic HP [5–8]. An identification of the culprit exposure is a pivotal step for adequate avoidance of the antigen, and there are several reports on the relationship between antigen identification and the clinical course of HP. Kypreos M et al. conducted a retrospective cohort study to evaluate whether the identification of antigens affects the clinical outcome in 136 fibrotic or nonfibrotic HP patients diagnosed in the ATS guidelines [9]. The result revealed that transplant-free survival was better in the patients where the antigens were identified. Pérez ERF et al. found that in the 142 patients diagnosed with chronic HP, survival was significantly longer in the patients with antigen identification [10].

The other reports also demonstrated the impact of antigen avoidance itself on the clinical course. Gimenez A et al. studied 112 cases of fibrotic HP and showed that approximately 40% of the cases in the antigen-avoidance group had sustained clinical improvement, which was significantly associated with lower mortality [5]. Petnak T et al. examined whether antigen identification and removal could predict all-cause mortality and lung transplantation rates in 377 fibrotic HP patients [6]. The results revealed that antigen identification and subsequent antigen avoidance were associated with decreased all-cause mortality and transplantation. Meaningfully, patients in whom a causative antigen was identified but who did not subsequently avoid exposure exhibited an increased risk of all-cause mortality and lung transplantation, comparable to that of patients in whom no antigen was identified. In a study of 121 fibrotic and nonfibrotic HP patients, Nishida et al. classified achievement of elimination of the causative antigen exposure into complete antigen avoidance (CAA) and inadequate antigen avoidance (IAA) [7]. As a result, all 30 nonfibrotic HP patients who achieved CAA showed no relapse or fibrosis progression, whereas 20 (45.5%) of the 44 with IAA had a relapse or fibrosis progression. As for the cases with fibrotic HP, there was a trend for IAA to be associated with decreased survival. Kawamoto et al. conducted a scoping review of 205 cases in 109 articles on HP and classified the achievement of antigen avoidance into four levels

[8]. The results concluded that patients who achieved adequate antigen avoidance were more likely to have good outcomes defined by "improvement/maintaining of the status."

Despite this evidence, there are still various challenges in accurately assessing the effectiveness of antigen avoidance as a treatment. First, it is difficult to prove whether the antigen that needs to be avoided is the true causative antigen. For example, it may be intricate to identify one specific antigen from the numerous antigens present in the environment that are frequently reported as causing HP. Conversely, the true causative antigen might have been overlooked due to the prominence of exposure to another antigen that is totally unrelated to the disease. Consequently, when the disease develops even after the antigen avoidance, it is difficult to determine whether treatment failure was due to insufficient antigen avoidance or to avoidance of a non-causative antigen. Second, the extent of antigen avoidance required for effective treatment is unclear. Namely, it is uncertain whether complete elimination of exposure is necessary or merely reducing exposure may be sufficient. This problem is particularly important when the causative antigen is widely present in our environment, such as birds or molds. Third, there is no way to evaluate how strictly patients adhere to antigen avoidance as instructed by their physicians.

There are also several barriers to carrying out antigen avoidance itself. Kawamoto et al. reported that inadequate antigen avoidance was due to financial constraints, lack of family cooperation, and professional reasons [8]. Aronson KI et al. established three discussion groups of ILD experts in the USA and identified the barriers to antigen identification and avoidance [11]. They found that the barriers to antigen identification included (1) unknown significance of the identified exposure antigen, (2) lack of knowledge on how to test for the suspected antigen, and (3) unavailability of the antigen of unknown cause.

Some cases of fibrotic HP may develop even after the antigen was avoided [12]. However, it remains unclear whether this phenomenon is due to insufficient antigen avoidance itself, or is based on the hypothesis that once the inflammatory reaction triggered by antigen exposure is turned on, it may persist even after antigen removal. For these reasons, accurate evaluation of the therapeutic effect of antigen avoidance remains a difficult proposition.

3 Antigen Avoidance in Practice

A comprehensive environmental survey is the first step of antigen avoidance. In the survey, the amount and duration of exposure are important factors to consider. For example, previous reports have demonstrated that the amount of antigen found in pigeon droppings in residential areas was significantly associated with a poor prognosis in patients with bird-related HP [13]. It is also known that housewives who spend a lot of time at home and are exposed to *Trichosporon* sp. are more likely to develop summer-type HP [14]. Therefore, the amount of antigen and the duration of exposure are important factors that can influence the incidence and prognosis of the disease. The use of a standardized questionnaire may be useful in identifying exposures. In order to gain a comprehensive understanding of the exposure, it is necessary to conduct the exposure assessment not only by a medical history but also by visits to the patient's home and workplace. Measurement of specific serum IgG antibodies is also useful for identifying the presence of exposure antigens that may be overlooked by medical history alone.

After exposure assessment was adequately implemented, the patients should make an effort to minimize their exposure to the causative antigen in their daily environments, including their homes, workplace, and hobbies. Patient education is crucial for successful antigen avoidance, as patients need to understand that fibrosis may continue to progress as long as they remain exposed to antigens, even after receiving treatment with corticosteroids or anti-fibrotic medications. Cooperation from patients, their families, and colleagues in the workplace is essential. Patient guidance should be clear, concise, and repeated. When renovation, relocation, or job changes become necessary, the financial and social burdens cannot be ignored. However, it is important to inform patients that if lung fibrosis progresses, medical costs and social burdens may increase in the future. If antigen avoidance is challenging for various reasons, strategies to reduce exposure, such as wearing masks and installing air purifiers, should be considered.

4 Avoidance for Individual Antigen

4.1 Bird-Related Hypersensitivity Pneumonitis (BRHP)

An avian antigen is the leading cause of fibrotic HP [15, 16]. Therefore, it is crucial to inquire about individuals' history of exposure to birds in their living environment. However, assessing the extent of exposure to avian antigens can be challenging, since bird-related hypersensitivity pneumonitis (BRHP) is caused not only by direct exposure such as the breeding of birds but also due to unrecognized exposure including feather products, wild birds, or breeding of birds by neighbors [17–22]. A previous report demonstrated a method for measuring the amount of avian antigen in an individual's environment. This report revealed that the amounts of avian antigen in household dust were associated with disease progression and a poor prognosis in patients with chronic bird-related HP [13]. From the same institution, Sema et al. presented a correlation between the mean amount of avian antigen and the decline of vital capacity over 1 year in patients with chronic BRHP [23].

To reduce exposure to avian antigens, contact with birds should be minimized. If birds are kept, it is recommended to discontinue breeding and remove the aviary. A previous report showed that high levels of avian antigens persisted for up to 18 months after removal [24], indicating that relocation is necessary in some cases. Down products, such as down quilts and jackets, should also be discarded. If poultry manure fertilizer has been used, it should be discontinued and properly disposed of, rather than stored in warehouses. Prohibiting agricultural activities alone is not sufficient to avoid exposure to the antigen. To further reduce exposure, it is desirable to avoid environments such as birdhouses or nests, bird feeding areas, locations where birds gather on walking trails, and situations where birds enter yards or balconies.

5 Summer-Type HP (SHP)

Summer-type hypersensitivity pneumonitis (SHP) is a type of home-related hypersensitivity pneumonitis that can result from exposure to fungi or molds present in the residential environment [25, 26]. *Trichosporon asahii* and *Trichosporon dermatitis* are specific antigens of SHP [27–29]. SHP typically manifests during the summer season when the growth of fungi or molds is prevalent. However, in recent years, SHP with winter onset has also been reported due to global warming, the spread of air conditioning systems, and the airtightness of buildings [30]. The disease has a relapse rate of 40% when antigen avoidance is inadequate. Therefore, the primary treatment for SHP typically involves relocation [14].

Some patients may be unable to relocate due to financial constraints or lack of motivation. In such cases, the removal of fungi or molds through renovation, house cleaning, disinfection, or alcohol use may be alternatives. Nevertheless, the effectiveness of these methods as a treatment for SHP is not well-supported. Yoshida K et al. conducted a study on 11 cases of SHP with various degrees of house cleaning [31]. The results revealed that none of the six patients who underwent thorough cleaning had a recurrence of SHP, whereas all patients living in homes that were either not cleaned or insufficiently cleaned developed recurrent disease. Inase et al. reported that among 10 cases of chronic SHP, those with persistent antigen exposure after diagnosis had a worse prognosis compared to those with improved environments through repair, renovation, or relocation [32]. Therefore, the effectiveness of antigen avoidance other than relocation depends on how thoroughly the removal of fungi or molds is carried out. Even if fungi or molds appear to be eliminated, they may remain within the walls or infiltrate from the exterior, rendering antigen avoidance inadequate, which needs careful observation.

6 Farmer's Lung

Thermophilic actinomycetes growing in dried grass are the causative antigens for farmer's lung, which is common among dairy livestock producers and greenhouse workers [33]. While a job change or workplace reassignment is ideal, there are several methods to reduce the antigen. It has been found that reducing the amount of antigens in stored grass can be achieved by drying or heating it. Placing the grass in round bales can be useful in preventing microbial growth. Additionally, slowing down the speed at which a silo is emptied or more strict ventilation in storage spaces are also considered [34–36].

7 Isocyanate-Induced Hypersensitivity Pneumonitis

The causative agent is isocyanate, which is released during car painting and spraying [37]. Generally, if exposure to isocyanates ceases, the prognosis is good [38], though there have been cases of exacerbation even after antigen avoidance [39], cases of ARDS [40], and cases of chronic progression requiring home oxygen therapy even after the use of prednisolone [41]. While complete antigen avoidance through workplace environmental improvement is necessary, the second best way is to lower the exposure concentration [42]. This may require improving work methods, modifying the workplace structure and ventilation, requiring employees to wear masks, and using protective equipment. The use of masks has already been shown to be effective [43], and the development of more protective masks is also underway.

8 Humidifier Lung

As the causative antigen is a microorganism that has proliferated in the humidifier [44], it is imperative to discontinue its use and dispose of the device. Humidifiers can be classified into three types: heated, vaporized, and ultrasonic. Of these, ultrasonic humidifiers are particularly susceptible to the growth of microorganisms and can easily become breeding grounds for bacteria and fungi. However, even other types of humidifiers can harbor microbial growth in their tray within a week's time [45]. Thus, it is important to avoid using humidifiers that have hard-to-clean tanks and to clean them regularly to minimize the risk of microbial growth.

9 Mushroom Worker's Lung

The HP observed in mushroom cultivators is known as "mushroom worker's lung" in Europe and has traditionally been attributed to thermophilic actinomycetes that grow in compost [46]. However, in recent years, reports of mushroom worker's lung caused by various types of mushrooms, such as shiitake, eryngii, and nameko, have been reported, and all of them have been attributed to inhalation of mushroom spores or the mushrooms themselves [47, 48]. Mushroom cultivators repeatedly inhale large amounts of airborne mushroom spores during the process of extracting strains from pots, known as "mushroom scratching," which causes the spores to become antigenic and results in the development of HP. Switching jobs or changing workplace assignments is the optimal solution, whereas the adequacy of wearing only a mask remains controversial. While one report presented that wearing only a mask was inadequate for disease control [49], several other reports have shown that patients were able to continue working while wearing N95 masks [47, 48].

10 Hot Tub Lung

Hot Tub Lung, a form of HP, has been reported to result from exposure to hot tubs, showers, and saunas [50]. The causative agent is the *Mycobacterium avium* complex (MAC), a nontuberculous mycobacterium that proliferates in stagnant water and is aerosolized by jet streams. It is important to note that MAC thrives at temperatures ranging from 25 to 30 °C, with a higher incidence during the summer months. However, cases of winter onset resulting from exposure to well water and hot water storage tank units have also been documented [51], indicating that MAC can occur throughout the year. Complete avoidance of exposure is critical for the treatment and many patients show well recovery only by antigen avoidance, while some severe cases had needed corticosteroid therapy [52, 53]. There is no adequate evidence to support antituberculous therapy being beneficial for the disease.

References

1. Selman M, Pardo A, King TE Jr. Hypersensitivity pneumonitis: insights in diagnosis and pathobiology. Am J Respir Crit Care Med. 2012;186(4):314–24.
2. Tsutsui T, Miyazaki Y, Okamoto T, et al. Antigen avoidance tests for diagnosis of chronic hypersensitivity pneumonitis. Respir Investig. 2015;53(5):217–24.
3. Okuda R, Takemura T, Iwasawa T, et al. Impact of antigen avoidance test for fibrotic hypersensitivity pneumonitis in stable phase. Allergy Asthma Clin Immunol. 2022;18(1):104.
4. Fernández Pérez ER, Travis WD, Lynch DA, et al. Diagnosis and evaluation of hypersensitivity pneumonitis: CHEST guideline and expert panel report. Chest. 2021;160:e97. https://doi.org/10.1016/j.chest.2021.03.066.
5. Gimenez A, Storrer K, Kuranishi L, Soares MR, Ferreira RG, Pereira CAC. Change in FVC and survival in chronic fibrotic hypersensitivity pneumonitis. Thorax. 2018;73(4):391–2.
6. Petnak T, Thongprayoon C, Baqir M, Ryu JH, Moua T. Antigen identification and avoidance on outcomes in fibrotic hypersensitivity pneumonitis. Eur Respir J. 2022;60:2101336. https://doi.org/10.1183/13993003.01336-2021.
7. Nishida T, Kawate E, Ishiguro T, Kanauchi T, Shimizu Y, Takayanagi N. Antigen avoidance and outcome of nonfibrotic and fibrotic hypersensitivity pneumonitis. ERJ Open Res. 2022;8(1) https://doi.org/10.1183/23120541.00474-2021.
8. Kawamoto Y, Oda S, Tanaka M. Antigen avoidance in people with hypersensitivity pneumonitis: a scoping review. Heart Lung. 2021;50(3):407–16. https://doi.org/10.1016/j.hrtlng.2021.01.023.
9. Kypreos M, Batra K, Glazer CS, Adams TN. Impact of number and type of identified antigen on transplant-free survival in hypersensitivity pneumonitis. PLoS One. 2022;17(9):e0273544.
10. Pérez ERF, Swigris JJ, Forssén AV, Tourin O. Identifying an inciting antigen is associated with improved survival in patients with chronic hypersensitivity pneumonitis. Chest. 2013; https://www.sciencedirect.com/science/article/pii/S0012369213607424
11. Aronson KI, O'Beirne R, Martinez FJ, Safford MM. Barriers to antigen detection and avoidance in chronic hypersensitivity pneumonitis in the United States. Respir Res. 2021;22(1):225.
12. Vasakova M, Morell F, Walsh S, Leslie K, Raghu G. Hypersensitivity pneumonitis: perspectives in diagnosis and management. Am J Respir Crit Care Med. 2017;196(6):680–9.

13. Tsutsui T, Miyazaki Y, Kuramochi J, Uchida K, Eishi Y, Inase N. The amount of avian antigen in household dust predicts the prognosis of chronic bird-related hypersensitivity pneumonitis. Ann Am Thorac Soc. 2015;12(7):1013–21.
14. Ando M, Arima K, Yoneda R, Tamura M. Japanese summer-type hypersensitivity pneumonitis. Geographic distribution, home environment, and clinical characteristics of 621 cases. Am Rev Respir Dis. 1991;144(4):765–9.
15. Morell F, Roger À, Reyes L, Cruz MJ, Murio C, Muñoz X. Bird fancier's lung: a series of 86 patients. Medicine. 2008;87(2):110–30.
16. Okamoto T, Miyazaki Y, Ogura T, et al. A nationwide epidemiological survey of chronic hypersensitivity pneumonitis in Japan. Respir Investig. 2013;51(3):191–9.
17. Greinert U, Lepp U, Becker W. Bird Keeper's lung without bird keepinge. Eur J Med Res. 2000;5(3):124.
18. Saltoun CA, Harris KE, Mathisen TL, Patterson R. Hypersensitivity pneumonitis resulting from community exposure to Canada goose droppings: when an external environmental antigen becomes an indoor environmental antigen. Ann Allergy Asthma Immunol. 2000;84(1):84–6.
19. Kokkarinen J, Tukiainen H, Seppä A, Terho EO. Hypersensitivity pneumonitis due to native birds in a bird ringer. Chest. 1994;106(4):1269–71.
20. Choy AC, Patterson R, Ray AH, Roberts M. Hypersensitivity pneumonitis in a raptor handler and a wild bird fancier. Ann Allergy Asthma Immunol. 1995;74(5):437–41.
21. Haitjema T, van Velzen-Blad H, van den Bosch JM. Extrinsic allergic alveolitis caused by goose feathers in a duvet. Thorax. 1992;47(11):990–1.
22. Inase N, Sakashita H, Ohtani Y, et al. Chronic bird fancier's lung presenting with acute exacerbation due to use of a feather duvet. Intern Med. 2004;43(9):835–7.
23. Sema M, Miyazaki Y, Tsutsui T, Tomita M, Eishi Y, Inase N. Environmental levels of avian antigen are relevant to the progression of chronic hypersensitivity pneumonitis during antigen avoidance. Immun Inflamm Dis. 2018;6(1):154–62.
24. Craig TJ, Hershey J, Engler RJ, Davis W, Carpenter GB, Salata K. Bird antigen persistence in the home environment after removal of the bird. Ann Allergy. 1992;69(6):510–2.
25. Selman M, Lacasse Y, Pardo A, Cormier Y. Hypersensitivity pneumonitis caused by fungi. Proc Am Thorac Soc. 2010;7(3):229–36.
26. Shimazu K, Ando M, Sakata T, Yoshida K, Araki S. Hypersensitivity pneumonitis induced by Trichosporon cutaneum. Am Rev Respir Dis. 1984;130(3):407–11.
27. Ando M, Suga M, Nishiura Y, Miyajima M. Summer-type hypersensitivity pneumonitis. Intern Med. 1995;34(8):707–12.
28. Kawai T, Tamura M, Murao M. Summer-type hypersensitivity pneumonitis. A unique disease in Japan. Chest. 1984;85(3):311–7.
29. Onishi Y, Kawamura T, Higashino T, Kagami R, Hirata N, Miyake K. Clinical features of chronic summer-type hypersensitivity pneumonitis and proposition of diagnostic criteria. Respir Investig. 2020;58(1):59–67.
30. Ishikawa T, Kawasaki T, Shimaya K, et al. Familial summer-type hypersensitivity pneumonitis induced in summer and winter at the work place. Arerugi. 2017;66(10):1236–9.
31. Yoshida K, Ando M, Sakata T, Araki S. Prevention of summer-type hypersensitivity pneumonitis: effect of elimination of Trichosporon cutaneum from the patients' homes. Arch Environ Health. 1989;44(5):317–22.
32. Inase N, Ohtani Y, Usui Y, Miyazaki Y, Takemura T, Yoshizawa Y. Chronic summer-type hypersensitivity pneumonitis: clinical similarities to idiopathic pulmonary fibrosis. Sarcoidosis Vasc Diffuse Lung Dis. 2007;24(2):141–7.
33. Cano-Jiménez E, Acuña A, Botana MI, et al. Farmer's lung disease. A review. Arch Bronconeumol. 2016;52(6):321–8.
34. Dalphin JC, Pernet D, Reboux G, et al. Influence of mode of storage and drying of fodder on thermophilic actinomycete aerocontamination in dairy farms of the Doubs region of France. Thorax. 1991;46(9):619–23.
35. Reboux G, Reiman M, Roussel S, et al. Impact of agricultural practices on microbiology of hay, silage and flour on Finnish and French farms. Ann Agric Environ Med. 2006;13(2):267–73.

36. Lange JL, Thorne PS, Lynch N. Application of flow cytometry and fluorescent in situ hybridization for assessment of exposures to airborne bacteria. Appl Environ Microbiol. 1997;63(4):1557–63.
37. Charles J, Bernstein A, Jones B, et al. Hypersensitivity pneumonitis after exposure to isocyanates. Thorax. 1976;31(2):127–36.
38. Saetta M, Maestrelli P, Di Stefano A, et al. Effect of cessation of exposure to toluene diisocyanate (TDI) on bronchial mucosa of subjects with TDI-induced asthma. Am Rev Respir Dis. 1992;145(1):169–74.
39. Akimoto T, Tamura N, Uchida K, Dambara T, Nukiwa T, Kira S. A case of hypersensitivity pneumonitis due to isocyanate exposure showing progression even two months after removal of the antigen. Nihon Kyobu Shikkan Gakkai Zasshi. 1992;30(3):458–63.
40. Morimatsu Y, Akiyoshi H, Tajiri M, Hirai R, Aizawa H. A case of hypersensitivity pneumonitis showing acute respiratory distress syndrome due to exposure to dust containing diphenylmethane diisocyanate. Nihon Kokyuki Gakkai Zasshi. 2004;42(6):502–8.
41. Nakamura Y, Fujimoto H, Uetani K, et al. A case of chronic hypersensitivity pneumonitis due to long term exposure to toluene diisocyanate. Nihon Kyobu Shikkan Gakkai Zasshi. 1995;33(4):429–32.
42. Kraw M, Tarlo SM. Isocyanate medical surveillance: respiratory referrals from a foam manufacturing plant over a five-year period. Am J Ind Med. 1999;35(1):87–91.
43. Hara S, Yamamoto K, Yoda A, et al. Three cases of isocyanate-induced hypersensitivity pneumonitis with different HRCT findings. Nihon Kokyuki Gakkai Zasshi. 2009;47(9):839–43.
44. Suda T, Sato A, Ida M, Gemma H, Hayakawa H, Chida K. Hypersensitivity pneumonitis associated with home ultrasonic humidifiers. Chest. 1995;107(3):711–7.
45. Onishi Y, Kawamura T, Tanaka H, et al. Evaluation of microorganisms of humidifier water and humidified air in home humidifier. Jpn J Sarcoidosis Other Granulomatous Disord. 2019;39(1_2):65–71.
46. Sakula A. Mushroom-worker's lung. Br Med J. 1967;3(5567):708–10.
47. Bringhurst LS, Byrne RN, Gershon-Cohen J. Respiratory disease of mushroom workers; farmer's lung. JAMA J Am Med Assoc. 1959;171:15–8.
48. Moore JE, Convery RP, Millar BC, Rao JR, Elborn JS. Hypersensitivity pneumonitis associated with mushroom worker's lung: an update on the clinical significance of the importation of exotic mushroom varieties. Int Arch Allergy Immunol. 2005;136(1):98–102.
49. Tsushima K, Furuya S, Yoshikawa S, et al. Therapeutic effects for hypersensitivity pneumonitis induced by Japanese mushroom (Bunashimeji). Am J Ind Med. 2006;49(10):826–35.
50. Fjällbrant H, Akerstrom M, Svensson E, Andersson E. Hot tub lung: an occupational hazard. Eur Respir Rev. 2013;22(127):88–90.
51. Sato N, Kawabata Y, Nagata M, Hagiwara K, Kanazawa M. A case of pulmonary Mycobacterium avium complex disease, mimicking hot tub lung. Nihon Kokyuki Gakkai Zasshi. 2006;44(12):962–7.
52. Hanak V, Kalra S, Aksamit TR, Hartman TE, Tazelaar HD, Ryu JH. Hot tub lung: presenting features and clinical course of 21 patients. Respir Med. 2006;100(4):610–5.
53. Griffith DE, Aksamit T, Brown-Elliott BA, et al. An official ATS/IDSA statement: diagnosis, treatment, and prevention of nontuberculous mycobacterial diseases. Am J Respir Crit Care Med. 2007;175(4):367–416.

Chapter 12
Steroid, Immunosuppressant, Anti-fibrotic Drug

How Much Does Steroid, Immunosuppressant, Anti-fibrotic Drug Contribute to Treatment and Prognosis?

Hiromi Tomioka

Abbreviation

BAL	Bronchoalveolar lavage
DLco	Carbon-monoxide-diffusing capacity
FEV1	Forced expiratory volume in 1 second
FVC	Forced vital capacity
HP	Hypersensitivity pneumonitis
IPF	Idiopathic pulmonary fibrosis
MMF	Mycophenolate mofetil
PF-ILD	Progressive fibrosing interstitial lung disease

1 Introduction

Antigen avoidance is critical for disease management of hypersensitivity pneumonitis (HP). However, there are cases where complete antigen avoidance is difficult or the causative antigen cannot be identified. Pharmacotherapy should then be considered in such scenarios, but currently, there are no evidence-based pharmacotherapy regimens for HP. Although the recent clinical practice guidelines [1, 2] address HP diagnosis, its pharmacological management was not comprehensively considered. These two guidelines [1, 2] updated the conventional categorization of acute, subacute, and chronic forms by classifying HP as either fibrotic or nonfibrotic. This

H. Tomioka (✉)
Department of Respiratory Medicine, Kobe City Medical Center West Hospital, Kobe, Japan
e-mail: htomy@kcho.jp

Y. Miyazaki (ed.), *Hypersensitivity Pneumonitis*, Respiratory Disease Series: Diagnostic Tools and Disease Managements,
https://doi.org/10.1007/978-981-96-7983-6_12

dichotomization seems to more closely correlate with both management considerations and overall prognosis.

Empirically, corticosteroids have been used as first-line therapy, and are effective in cases of nonfibrotic HP with acute onset; they have short-term effects in improving symptoms during the acute phase but long-term improvement has been rarely reported. Considering the limitations of corticosteroid therapy, other anti-inflammatory and immunosuppressive treatments have been applied for fibrotic HP. Moreover, because fibrotic HP and idiopathic pulmonary fibrosis (IPF) seem to share common pathogenetic mechanisms [3–5], there is accumulating evidence that antifibrotic medications can be useful as second-line therapy in some patients with fibrotic HP who progress despite anti-inflammatory and immunosuppressive treatments [6, 7].

2 Corticosteroids

In a prospective study of 93 patients with farmer's lung treated with corticosteroid either for 4 weeks, 12 weeks, or not at all, early symptom improvement was reported in those patients receiving the drug [8]. However, no differences were apparent regarding symptoms and respiratory function in the long term. In another study, a randomized, placebo-controlled trial in the early 1990s tested an 8-week tapering course of corticosteroid (prednisolone) including 36 patients with farmer's lung [9]. After one month of treatment, significant differences in the carbon-monoxide-diffusing capacity (DLco) between treated and untreated patients were noted, but on long-term follow-up, no statistically significant differences were found in the forced vital capacity (FVC), forced expiratory volume in 1 s (FEV1), or DLco at 5 years. A retrospective study [10] using linear mixed-effect modeling of changes in respiratory function attributed to corticosteroid treatment examined 67 patients with non-fibrotic HP treated with corticosteroids. In that study, a significant increase in %FVC and a tendency toward improvement in %DLco was observed. However, in another study of 82 patients with fibrotic HP, no significant changes were observed in either %FVC or %DLco on treatment with corticosteroids. In addition, a comparison of 109 cases of fibrotic HP, treated or not treated with corticosteroids, revealed no differences in survival. In a single-center retrospective study [11] conducted to investigate whether the presence of bronchoalveolar lavage (BAL) lymphocytosis (>20%) or honeycombing on CT influenced the effect of corticosteroid treatment of fibrotic HP patients, both a low degree of BAL lymphocytosis and honeycombing predicted a lack of treatment efficacy and a poor outcome. In contrast, a marginal increase in FVC was recorded in patients with high BAL lymphocytosis or the absence of honeycombing.

In a comparative study of fibrotic HP in 30 corticosteroid-treated or untreated patients in a propensity score-matched cohort [12], the survival rate was significantly better for those treated, and absolute values of the FVC after 6, 12, and 24 months showed significant improvement. This was the first report to document a survival benefit associated with corticosteroid treatment of patients with fibrotic HP. This suggests that even in patients with fibrotic HP, those with mild-to-moderate fibrosis and evidence of ground-glass opacities could still be a promising target population for treatment with corticosteroids. A parallel comparative prospective trial assessed the effect of corticosteroid treatment (0.5 mg/kg/day of methylprednisolone for 8 weeks) in both fibrotic HP ($n = 21$) and nonfibrotic HP ($n = 32$) [13]. A significantly better improvement in clinical and functional status was reported in patients with nonfibrotic relative to fibrotic HP. Nonetheless, there was still a significant improvement in FEV1, FVC, oximetry, and six-minute walk test in fibrotic HP patients after corticosteroid treatment.

3 Other Anti-inflammatory and Immunosuppressive Drugs

The frequently progressive nature of HP, despite corticosteroid treatment, as well as their serious side effects, has promoted an active search for other effective anti-inflammatory and immunosuppressive drugs. A retrospective study of 59 patients treated with azathioprine for 1 year found that BAL lymphocytosis in 36 of the patients was associated with a response to treatment [14]. In a retrospective study of 62 patients with chronic HP who also received azathioprine [15], 35 continued treatment for 2 years and exhibited significant improvements in the FVC but not DLco at 12 and 24 months. In contrast, in another retrospective study of 70 patients with chronic HP who received mycophenolate mofetil (MMF) or azathioprine [16], there was no significant effect on %FVC, but this time significant improvement of %DLco after 1 year was reported. A further retrospective study of 30 patients with chronic HP treated with MMF or azathioprine [17] documented that in the 22 who continued treatment for 1 year (18 on MMF, 4 on azathioprine), a significant improvement in DLco was achieved and dose reduction of corticosteroids became possible. Another study of 93 patients with chronic HP, 41 of whom were treated with corticosteroid monotherapy and 52 with MMF or azathioprine combination therapy [18], found that FVC decline and survival were similar between the two treatment groups; however, patients receiving the combination therapy reported less treatment-emergent adverse events. A retrospective study sought factors predicting treatment success and survival advantage in 93 HP patients treated with corticosteroids alone or in combination with azathioprine [19]. Among those with fibrotic HP ($n = 54$), improvement was noted in 19 (35%) cases. A multivariate analysis showed that only the presence of fibrosis in high-resolution CT remained a significant factor associated with negative treatment outcome.

Because a recent investigation reported that telomere length may influence the response to immunosuppressive drugs, including MMF [20], an observational study assessed the influence of MMF on chronic HP outcomes using telomere length measurement [21]. MMF therapy was not associated with improved survival or lung function in patients with chronic HP and short telomeres. In contrast, in the absence of such short telomeres, improved survival was associated with MMF in chronic

HP. Telomere length may thus represent a biomarker to identify patients with fibrotic HP at risk of poor outcomes when immunosuppressed.

The tolerability and effectiveness of leflunomide, a derivative of isoxazole used as a disease-modifying antirheumatic drug, was evaluated in 40 patients with chronic HP [22]. Significant increments in %FVC and %DLco were observed in nonfibrotic HP with 20% or less fibrosis on CT; however, no improvement was observed for fibrotic HP with >20% fibrosis. The corticosteroid dose could be reduced for 31 patients who were receiving corticosteroids at the start of leflunomide treatment, and could be completely discontinued within 1 year for 12 patients. Leflunomide should be used with caution, however, because fatal lung injury became a problem soon after its launch in Japan, and pre-existing interstitial lung disease is considered the most important risk factor for leflunomide-induced lung injury [23].

A retrospective study of 20 patients with chronic HP who did not improve despite antigen avoidance and corticosteroid therapy reported that treatment with rituximab, an anti-CD20 monoclonal antibody, showed some benefit [24]. FVC decreased for all cases in the 6 months preceding the introduction of rituximab, but it improved or stabilized in 7 of them (35%) after 6 months of antibody administration; DLco improved in 5 of 8 patients (63%) for whom this parameter was measured. A significant reduction in the corticosteroid dose was also possible. However, 7 patients (35%) developed an infection, and one died from respiratory infection.

Despite the relative lack of high-quality evidence, it is clear that some patients, even those with fibrotic HP, particularly those with a greater degree of active inflammation, experience significant benefit from anti-inflammatory and immunosuppressive therapies. Table 12.1 summarizes factors associated with these treatment outcomes in HP.

Table 12.1 Factors associated with anti-inflammatory/immunosuppressive treatment outcomes in hypersensitivity pneumonitis

Factor	Study population	Pharmacotherapy	Outcomes	References
BAL lymphocytosis	Fibrotic HP	Corticosteroids	10-year survival	[11]
BAL lymphocytosis	Chronic HP	Azathioprine	Disease stabilization	[14]
Honeycombing on CT	Fibrotic HP	Corticosteroids	10-year survival	[11]
Fibrosis on HRCT	Fibrotic and nonfibrotic HP	Corticosteroids ± azathioprine	Treatment outcomes[a]	[19]
Telomere length	Chronic HP	Mycophenolate mofetil	Transplant-free survival	[21]
Significant fibrosis on CT	Chronic HP	Leflunomide	FVC, DLco	[22]

BAL Bronchoalveolar lavage, *DLco* carbon-monoxide-diffusing capacity, *FVC* forced vital capacity, *HRCT* high-resolution CT

[a]Treatment outcomes are classified as improvement, stable disease, and progression based on a combination of pulmonary function tests and chest X-ray

4 Antifibrotic Drugs

A randomized placebo-controlled trial of 663 patients with progressive fibrosing interstitial lung diseases other than IPF (26.1% with HP) using the antifibrotic drug nintedanib, which is approved for the treatment of IPF, demonstrated significant suppression of the annual rate of decline in FVC [6]. The indication for "Progressive Fibrosing Interstitial Lung Disease" (PF-ILD) or "Chronic Fibrosing Interstitial Lung Diseases with a Progressive Phenotype" was therefore also approved for this drug. In a subgroup analysis based on ILD diagnosis [25], HP with PF-ILD patients exhibited characteristics similar to the overall population, suggesting that nintedanib might be effective here too.

Pirfenidone, another antifibrotic drug, is also being studied for its efficacy against fibrotic (chronic) HP. In a retrospective study of 23 patients with chronic HP [26], the vital capacity in the 6 months following the start of treatment was significantly improved relative to the 6 months before treatment. An open-label comparative study of chronic HP involving 9 patients receiving corticosteroids plus azathioprine and 13 patients receiving corticosteroids plus azathioprine and pirfenidone [27] concluded that after 1 year of treatment, there was no difference in the FVC. However, a marginal improvement in the DLco and a significant improvement in the health-related quality of life were reported for the patients also receiving pirfenidone. A phase 2 trial (RELIEF) in PF-ILD patients (excluding IPF) with an annual decline of %FVC of at least 5% despite conventional therapy showed a significantly slower decline in %FVC in those receiving pirfenidone relative to placebo [7]. The most frequent diagnosis of ILD was chronic HP with 57 cases (45%). However, considering that the study was terminated prematurely, these results should be interpreted with caution. In a retrospective study of 30 patients with fibrotic HP who continued antifibrotic drug monotherapy (14 pirfenidone, 16 nintedanib) [28], a significant annual decline in %FVC and %DLco over a period of 3 years was reported nonetheless. In future, the treatment strategy for fibrotic HP will likely shift to combination therapies with anti-inflammatory/ immunosuppressive and antifibrotic drugs.

5 Pharmacotherapy Strategy in Clinical Practice

Figure 12.1 illustrates the treatment algorithm based on the recently published Japanese clinical practice guide for HP [29].

- Nonfibrotic HP that includes acute HP.

Corticosteroid treatment is indicated when antigen avoidance is not possible or for patients with respiratory failure. Prednisolone should be started at a dose of 0.5–1.0 mg/kg/day. If hypoxemia is severe, pulse therapy with corticosteroid (methylprednisolone 0.5–1 g/day for 3 days) should be started, followed by prednisolone at a dose of 0.5–1.0 mg/kg/day. No consensus exists on the tapering procedure or

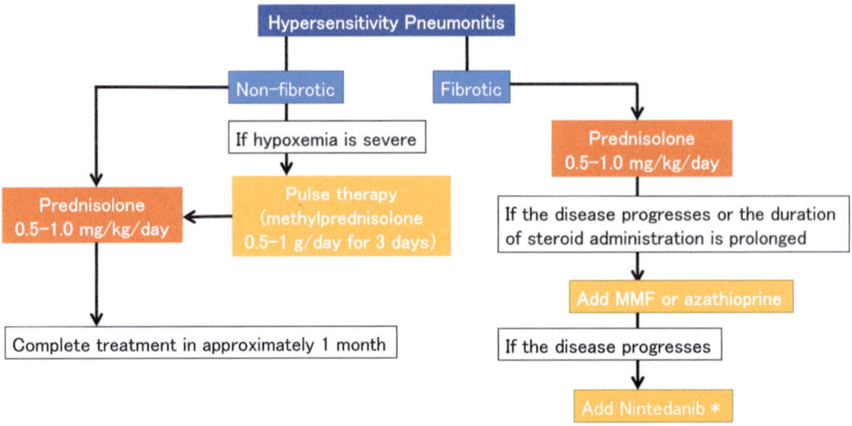

Fig. 12.1 Pharmacotherapy strategy algorithm for hypersensitivity pneumonitis. MMF mycophenolate mofetil. *When the radiological or pathological findings are consistent with usual interstitial pneumonia pattern, the corticosteroid dose should be reduced and antifibrotic drugs should be considered as the main treatment

duration of treatment; however, the goal should be to complete treatment in approximately 1 month.

- Fibrotic HP.

Prednisolone should be started at a dose of 0.5–1.0 mg/kg/day. No consensus exists on the tapering procedure or duration of treatment, and the prednisolone dose should be tapered while monitoring clinical symptoms, respiratory function, and imaging findings. If the disease progresses or the duration of steroid administration is prolonged, MMF or azathioprine should be added to the regimen, and the corticosteroid should be tapered off. Nintedanib should be administered if the clinical course of the disease is consistent with PF-ILD. When the radiological or pathological findings are consistent with usual interstitial pneumonia pattern, the corticosteroids dose should be reduced and antifibrotic drugs should be considered as the main treatment from the perspective of the toxicity of anti-inflammatories for IPF [30].

Conflict of Interest Hiromi Tomioka received lecture fees from Nippon Boehringer Ingelheim Co., Ltd.

References

1. Raghu G, Remy-Jardin M, Ryerson CJ, Myers JL, Kreuter M, Vasakova M, et al. Diagnosis of hypersensitivity pneumonitis in adults. An official ATS/JRS/ALAT clinical practice guideline. Am J Respir Crit Care Med. 2020;202:e36–69.
2. Fernández Pérez ER, Travis WD, Lynch DA, Brown KK, Johannson KA, Selman M, et al. Executive summary: diagnosis and evaluation of hypersensitivity pneumonitis: CHEST guideline and expert panel report. Chest. 2021;160:595–615.

3. Jinta T, Miyazaki Y, Kishi M, Akashi T, Takemura T, Inase N, et al. The pathogenesis of chronic hypersensitivity pneumonitis in common with idiopathic pulmonary fibrosis: expression of apoptotic markers. Am J Clin Pathol. 2010;134:613–20.
4. García de Alba C, Buendia-Roldán I, Salgado A, Becerril C, Ramírez R, González Y, et al. Fibrocytes contribute to inflammation and fibrosis in chronic hypersensitivity pneumonitis through paracrine effects. Am J Respir Crit Care Med. 2015;191:427–36.
5. Ley B, Newton CA, Arnould I, Elicker BM, Henry TS, Vittinghoff E, et al. The MUC5B promoter polymorphism and telomere length in patients with chronic hypersensitivity pneumonitis: an observational cohort-control study. Lancet Respir Med. 2017;5:639–47.
6. Flaherty KR, Wells AU, Cottin V, Devaraj A, Walsh SLF, Inoue Y, et al. Nintedanib in progressive fibrosing interstitial lung diseases. N Engl J Med. 2019;381:1718–27.
7. Behr J, Prasse A, Kreuter M, Johow J, Rabe KF, Bonella F, et al. Pirfenidone in patients with progressive fibrotic interstitial lung diseases other than idiopathic pulmonary fibrosis(RELIEF): a double-blind, randomised, placebo-controlled, phase 2b trial. Lancet Respir Med. 2021;9:476–86.
8. Mönkäre S. Influence of corticosteroid treatment on the course of farmer's lung. Eur J Respir Dis. 1983;64:283–93.
9. Kokkarinen JI, Tukiainen HO, Terho EO. Effect of corticosteroid treatment on the recovery of pulmonary function in farmer's lung. Am Rev Respir Dis. 1992;145:3–5.
10. De Sadeleer LJ, Hermans F, De Dycker E, et al. Effects of corticosteroid treatment and antigen avoidance in a large hypersensitivity pneumonitis cohort: a single-centre cohort study. J Clin Med. 2018;8:14.
11. De Sadeleer LJ, Hermans F, De Dycker E, Yserbyt J, Verschakelen JA, Verbeken EK, et al. Impact of BAL lymphocytosis and presence of honeycombing on corticosteroid treatment effect in fibrotic hypersensitivity pneumonitis: a retrospective cohort study. Eur Respir J. 2020;55:1901983.
12. Ejima M, Okamoto T, Suzuki T, Anzai T, Takahashi K, Miyazaki Y. Efficacy of treatment with corticosteroids for fibrotic hypersensitivity pneumonitis: a propensity score-matched cohort analysis. BMC Pulm Med. 2021;21:243.
13. Tony FA, Soliman YMA, Salem HA. Effect of oral methyl prednisolone on different radiological patterns of hypersensitivity pneumonitis. J Asthma Allergy. 2021;14:501–11.
14. Raimundo S, Pimenta AC, Cruz-Martins N, Rodrigues MC, Melo N, Mota PC, et al. Insights on chronic hypersensitivity pneumonitis' treatment: factors associated with a favourable response to azathioprine. Life Sci. 2021;272:119274.
15. Terras Alexandre A, Martins N, Raimundo S, Melo N, Catetano Mota P, Novais E, Bastos H, et al. Impact of azathioprine use in chronic hypersensitivity pneumonitis patients. Pulm Pharmacol Ther. 2020;60:101878.
16. Morisset J, Johannson KA, Vittinghoff E, Aravena C, Elicker BM, Jones KD, et al. Use of mycophenolate mofetil or azathioprine for the management of chronic hypersensitivity pneumonitis. Chest. 2017;151:619–25.
17. Fiddler CA, Simler N, Thillai M, Parfrey H. Use of mycophenolate mofetil and azathioprine for the treatment of chronic hypersensitivity pneumonitis-A single-centre experience. Clin Respir J. 2019;13:791–4.
18. Adegunsoye A, Oldham JM, Fernández Pérez ER, Hamblin M, Patel N, Tener M, et al. Outcomes of immunosuppressive therapy in chronic hypersensitivity pneumonitis. ERJ Open Res. 2017;3:00016–2017.
19. Lewandowska KB, Barańska I, Sobiecka M, Radwan-Rohrenschef P, Dybowska M, Franczuk M, et al. Factors predictive for immunomodulatory therapy response and survival in patients with hypersensitivity pneumonitis-retrospective cohort analysis. Diagnostics (Basel). 2022;12:2767.
20. Newton CA, Zhang D, Oldham JM, Kozlitina J, Ma SF, Martinez FJ, et al. Telomere length and use of immunosuppressive medications in idiopathic pulmonary fibrosis. Am J Respir Crit Care Med. 2019;200:336–47.

21. Adegunsoye A, Morisset J, Newton CA, Oldham JM, Vittinghoff E, Linderholm AL, et al. Leukocyte telomere length and mycophenolate therapy in chronic hypersensitivity pneumonitis. Eur Respir J. 2021;57:2002872.
22. Noh S, Yadav R, Li M, Wang X, Sahoo D, Culver DA, et al. Use of leflunomide in patients with chronic hypersensitivity pneumonitis. BMC Pulm Med. 2020;20:199.
23. Sawada T, Inokuma S, Sato T, Otsuka T, Saeki Y, Takeuchi T, et al. Leflunomide-induced interstitial lung disease: prevalence and risk factors in Japanese patients with rheumatoid arthritis. Rheumatology (Oxford). 2009;48:1069–72.
24. Ferreira M, Borie R, Crestani B, Rigaud P, Wemeau L, Israel-Biet D, et al. Efficacy and safety of rituximab in patients with chronic hypersensitivity pneumonitis (cHP): a retrospective, multicentric, observational study. Respir Med. 2020;172:106146.
25. Wells AU, Flaherty KR, Brown KK, Inoue Y, Devaraj A, Richeldi L, et al. Nintedanib in patients with progressive fibrosing interstitial lung diseases-subgroup analyses by interstitial lung disease diagnosis in the INBUILD trial: a randomised, double-blind, placebo-controlled, parallel-group trial. Lancet Respir Med. 2020;8:453–60.
26. Shibata S, Furusawa H, Inase N. Pirfenidone in chronic hypersensitivity pneumonitis: a real-life experience. Sarcoidosis Vasc Diffuse Lung Dis. 2018;35:139–42.
27. Mateos-Toledo H, Mejía-Ávila M, Rodríguez-Barreto Ó, Mejía-Hurtado JG, Rojas-Serrano J, Estrada A, et al. An open-label study with pirfenidone on chronic hypersensitivity pneumonitis. Arch Bronconeumol (Engl Ed). 2020;56:163–9.
28. Tzilas V, Tzouvelekis A, Bouros E, Karampitsakos T, Ntassiou M, Avdoula E, et al. Clinical experience with antifibrotics in fibrotic hypersensitivity pneumonitis: a 3-year real-life observational study. ERJ Open Res. 2020;6:00152–2020.
29. Tomioka H, Miyazaki Y, Inoue Y, Egashira R, Kawamura T, Sano H, et al. Japanese clinical practice guide 2022 for hypersensitivity pneumonitis. Respir Investig. 2024;62(1):16–43.
30. Idiopathic Pulmonary Fibrosis Clinical Research Network, Raghu G, Anstrom KJ, King TE Jr, Lasky JA, Martinez FJ. Prednisone, azathioprine, and N-acetylcysteine for pulmonary fibrosis. N Engl J Med. 2012;366:1968–77.

Part IV
Individual Hypersensitivity Pneumonitis

Chapter 13
Summer-Type Hypersensitivity Pneumonitis

What Is Summer-Type Hypersensitivity Pneumonitis?

Tetsuji Kawamura

1 Summer-Type Hypersensitivity Pneumonitis as a Disease Entity

Hypersensitivity pneumonitis (HP) that worsens in the summer was first described around 1973, and this interesting form of HP was named "summer-type hypersensitivity pneumonitis" (SHP) in 1978 by Miyagawa et al. [1]. According to a 1980 Ministry of Health and Welfare study group report, most cases of HP in Japan were SHP, and the causative antigen was *Cryptococcus*.

However, a later study found that the main causative antigen of SHP was *Tricosporon cutaneum* [2]. *T. cutaneum* was detected in the patient's house [3], precipitating antibody for *T. cutaneum* was present [4], and an inhalation challenge test [5] was positive. In 1991, Ando et al. [6] reported 621 cases of SHP and concluded that the main causative antigen was *T. cutaneum*. From the microbiological examination of the house of patients with SHP, three serotypes of *Tricosporon* species, including *T. dermatis* (*T. mucoides*), *T. asahii*, and *T. montevideen*, are considered to be the causative antigens of SHP [7]. The classification of *Trichosporon* species was changed based on gene analyses of the *Trichosporon* genus, and *T. cutaneum* was reclassified as *T. asahii* and others. In a study of patients with anti-*T. asahii* antibody-positive SHP, *T. asahii* nucleic acid was found in the broncheoalveolar lavage fluid (BALF) of patients, suggesting that *T. asahii* was the most common causative antigen of SHP [8].

Currently, in Japan, an enzyme-linked immunosorbent assay for anti-*T. asahii* antibody is the only commercially available quantitative assay for measuring

T. Kawamura (✉)
Department of Respiratory Medicine, National Hospital Organization Himeji Medical Center, Himeji City, Japan

Y. Miyazaki (ed.), *Hypersensitivity Pneumonitis*, Respiratory Disease Series: Diagnostic Tools and Disease Managements,
https://doi.org/10.1007/978-981-96-7983-6_13

antibodies to *Trichosporon* species, making it difficult to diagnose SHP caused by *Trichosporon* species other than *T. asahii*.

2 Acute (Nonfibrotic) Summer Hypersensitivity Pneumonitis

2.1 Epidemiology

According to a national investigation conducted from 1980 to 1989, 621 of 835 HP cases (74.4%) were SHP, of which 85.7% of cases developed from June to September, and the peak was in July [6]. Of the patients with SHP, 89.5% lived in wooden houses, and the mean age of the building was 20.5 years. More than half the houses had unsanitary conditions such as shady, damp, or poorly ventilated rooms. The age of onset ranged from 2 to 86 years (peak in the 40 s). The number of female patients was double that of male patients, and 39.8% were full-time homemakers. The rates of family-onset cases and smoking among male and female patients were 23.8%, 61.4%, and 5.3%, respectively.

In a review of 25 families and 50 cases of familial SHP in Japan, all familial occurrences of SHP occurred within 2 months of the first case of HP within the family, and eight of the 23 (35%) family members studied were not blood relatives of the index case in the family. Additionally, 28 of the 50 (56%) of patients with SHP were women, and four of the 31 (13%) family members studied were current smokers. The incidence of HP among women homemakers and nonsmokers was relatively high. Furthermore, 25 of 50 (50%) patients received steroid therapy, and the other 50% improved without medication. Additionally, 19 of the 47 (40%) patients moved to another residence [9].

Many SHP cases resolved spontaneously without treatment in November, and 38% of the cases that resolved spontaneously recurred the following summer. In Japan, the rainy season from June to mid-July is followed by a hot and humid summer season. Because *Trichosporon* species grow well at temperatures of 25–28 °C and 80% humidity, they grow easily in wooden houses during the rainy season in Japan. Therefore, the incidence of SHP is high in the western and southern regions of Japan [10], and a case of SHP has been reported on the nearby Jeju Island of South Korea [11].

According to a land statistics survey by the Ministry of Internal Affairs and Communications Statistics Bureau, the proportion of wooden construction in Japan decreased from 73.0% in 1988 to 58.9% in 2008. Global warming, increased airtightness of houses, increased use of air conditioners, and decreased smoking rates may have contributed to changes in the SHP incidence rate.

2.2 *Symptoms, Physical Examination, and Laboratory Findings, HRCT Findings*

Common symptoms of SHP include cough in almost all cases, exertional dyspnea in 90%, and fever in 80% of patients. Physical examination reveals fine inspiratory crackles. Laboratory findings reveal leukopenia, elevated levels of C-reactive protein, and hypoxemia [6, 10]. Increases in Krebs von den Lungen-6 (KL-6) and blood surfactant protein-D (SP-D) levels are higher than those observed in other interstitial lung diseases [12].

Pulmonary function tests reveal a decrease in vital capacity and diffusion capacity, and sometimes obstructive disorders. BALF reveals lymphocytosis and a decrease in the CD 4/8 ratio [6, 10, 13]. High-resolution computed tomography (HRCT) reveals ground-glass opacities, mosaic attenuation, ill-defined centrilobular nodules, and air trapping in the expiratory phase (Fig. 13.1). Pathological findings reveal cellular interstitial pneumonia, cellular bronchiolitis, and poorly formed nonnecrotizing granulomas [14].

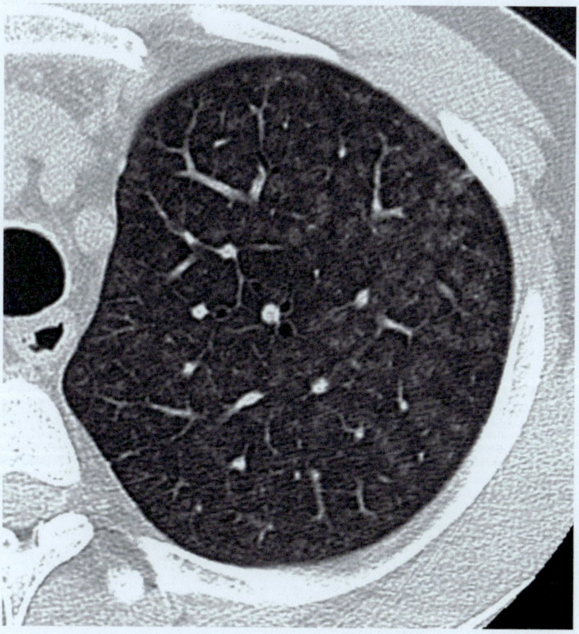

Fig. 13.1 High-resolution computed tomography findings of a case of acute (nonfibrotic) summer-type hypersensitivity pneumonitis. High-resolution computed tomography in a 51-year-old man showing diffuse, hazy, and small nodules. The patient had no history of smoking and had October-onset anti-*Trichosporon asahii* antibody positivity. Bronchoalveolar lavage revealed lymphocytosis (88%), and transbronchial biopsy revealed alveolitis, granulomas, and organizing pneumonia. The patient's symptoms improved after environmental rehabilitation of his house

2.3 Diagnosis

A definite diagnosis of acute SHP requires positive results for anti-*T. asahii* antibody and specific findings on HRCT [14, 15]. Even if the anti-*T. asahii* antibody is negative or nonmeasurable, the diagnosis of acute SHP is possible when there is a relationship among its onset, circumstances (e.g., summer onset, exacerbation at home, remission by avoidance of the causative antigen), and specific histopathological findings. The diagnosis of SHP caused by *Trichosporon* species other than *T. asahii* is performed similarly as the *T. asahii* antibody-positive cases.

The symptoms are relieved after hospitalization for a few days or several weeks, and recur after 4–8 h of returning to the home, at a rate of 91.4% [6]; therefore, the circumstance-provocation test is useful. When the symptoms or various findings of SHP improve after avoidance of the causative antigen, the patient returns home and stays for one or a few days. If elevations in body temperature, leukocyte count, C-reactive protein levels, or alveolar-arterial oxygen difference (A-aDO_2); exacerbation of pulmonary function; or HRCT findings are observed, the provocation test is positive. Acute SHP is the most common type of HP in Japan, and simple diagnostic criteria have been proposed (Table 13.1).

2.4 Prognosis and Treatment

The prognosis is good for patients in the early stages with antigen avoidance [10]. However, if the causative antigen cannot be avoided, the symptoms and pulmonary function gradually aggravate by progressive pulmonary fibrosis. The removal of the *Trichosporon* antigen from the home environment is the most important step. This can be achieved by moving into a new house or refurbishing the existing house [16]. When adequate antigen removal is not possible, corticosteroids may be administered after informing the patient of their long-term side effects [3].

Table 13.1 Diagnostic criteria of acute (nonfibrotic) summer-type hypersensitivity pneumonitis

Clinical items
1. Onset in summer (from May to October) with cough, dyspnea, and fever
2. Typical high-resolution computed tomography findings for nonfibrotic HP
3. Positive for anti-*Trichosporon asahii* antibody
4. A positive provocation test (exacerbation at home)
5. (a) Lymphocytosis in bronchoalveolar lavage fluid, or
(b) Typical pathological findings for nonfibrotic HP diagnosis
(1), (2), (3), and (4) and/or (5); Nonfibrotic SHP induced by *T. asahii*
(1), (2), and (4); Nonfibrotic SHP of unknown etiology
(1), (2), and (5); Probable nonfibrotic SHP of unknown etiology
If the cause is identified, a diagnosis of nonfibrotic SHP is made.

Abbreviations: *HP* hypersensitivity pneumonitis, *SHP* summer-type hypersensitivity pneumonitis

3 Chronic (Fibrotic) Summer Hypersensitivity Pneumonitis

3.1 Epidemiology

The diagnosis of chronic (fibrotic) SHP is more difficult than that of acute (nonfibrotic) SHP, because it is difficult to confirm environment-induced exacerbation or improvement by avoidance of the causative antigen. Although cases of bird-related chronic HP have been reported worldwide, most cases of chronic SHP have been reported from Japan, and knowledge of its epidemiology is limited.

In 1999, Yoshizawa et al. [17] reported the results of a national investigation on chronic hypersensitivity pneumonitis (CHP), conducted in Japan. The study described ten cases of chronic SHP (28%) among 36 cases of CHP. As acute SHP is the most common type of acute HP, this finding was unexpected.

3.2 Diagnosis

In the CHEST guideline [15], the probability of the causative antigen is classified as "identified," "indeterminate," or "unidentified," and a flowchart for diagnosis is provided for each of these classifications. Because the cutoff level of the *T. asahii* antibody has not been defined, and the results of environment-provocation tests are often unclear in patients with chronic SHP, the probability of the causative antigen is "indeterminate" in many cases. Therefore, for a diagnosis of chronic SHP, at least two of three of the following criteria are required: (1) characteristic HRCT findings (Fig. 13.2); (2) BALF lymphocytosis; and (3) characteristic histopathological findings in a surgical lung biopsy. However, the cutoff level of BALF lymphocyte percentage in the diagnosis of chronic SHP has not been defined, and surgical lung biopsy is sometimes dangerous and often difficult in patients with severe pulmonary fibrosis. Thus, less-invasive diagnostic criteria for chronic SHP have been suggested [18], including (1) anti-*T. asahii* antibody positivity; (2) HRCT patterns consistent with FHP, including mosaic attenuation or micronodules; and (3) elevated serum biomarker levels (KL-6 > 1500 U/mL or SP-D > 250 ng/mL). Cases satisfying criteria (1) and (2) are defined as "probable fibrotic SHP," and those satisfying all three criteria as "confident clinical diagnosis of fibrotic SHP."

Although use of the antigen avoidance test during 2-week hospitalization has been proposed for the diagnosis of chronic SHP, the improvement trend after avoidance has not shown a statistically significant difference, and further investigation is necessary [19].

Differentiation of chronic SHP from idiopathic interstitial pneumonias (IIPs) is important. Inase et al. [20] reported 14 cases of chronic SHP and noted similarities to idiopathic pulmonary fibrosis (IPF). In this study, specific antibodies against *T. asahii* and *T. mucoides* were positive in sera and BALF of 12 of 14 patients with chronic SHP, and the lymphocyte proliferation test induced by *Trichosporon*-related antigen was positive in all five patients tested. Traction bronchiectasis and honeycombing on HRCT were observed in more than 70% of cases.

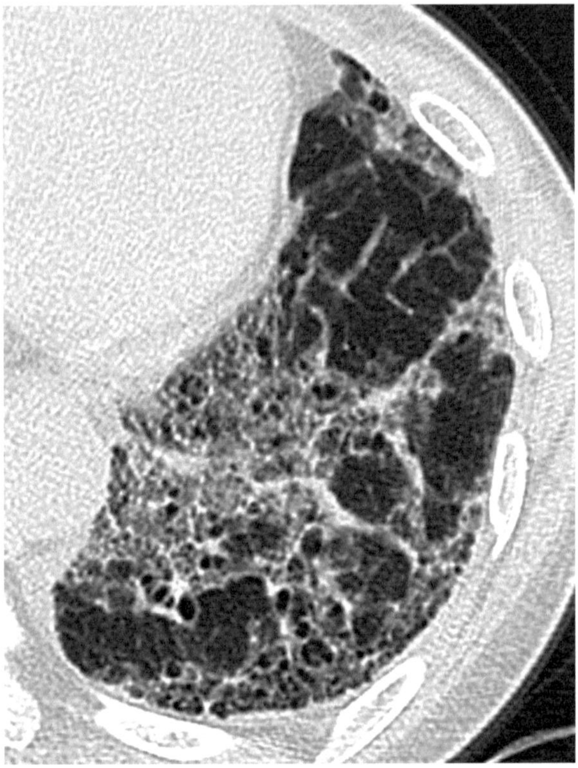

Fig. 13.2 High-resolution computed tomography findings of a case of chronic (fibrotic) summer-type hypersensitivity pneumonitis. High-resolution computed tomography in a 60-year-old woman showing diffuse centrilobular nodules and fibrotic changes with a mosaic pattern. The patient had no history of smoking and was anti-*Trichosporon asahii* antibody positive. Bronchoalveolar lavage revealed mild lymphocytosis (28%), and surgical lung biopsy revealed a usual interstitial pneumonia-like pattern with centrilobular fibrosis. The patient's symptoms improved slightly after environmental rehabilitation of her house

In another report by the same group, two cases of chronic SHP misdiagnosed as IIPs were described in detail [21]. Both cases were *Trichosporon* antibody-positive (in one case, *T. mucoides* was detected in the home) and had honeycombing of the lungs on HRCT, which is characteristic of IPF. However, the histopathological findings of the autopsy revealed pulmonary fibrosis in the centrilobular and perilobular areas, which is compatible with fibrotic HP.

Future studies should address the following three questions: (1) setting a cutoff level of the anti-*T. asahii* antibody for the diagnosis of chronic SHP, (2) developing commercial measurement of antibodies to microorganisms other than *T. asahii*, and (3) developing a practical method of conducting antigen-avoidance testing for the diagnosis of chronic SHP.

3.3 Prognosis and Treatment

In the above study, three of the four patients who did not remedy their houses died, suggesting a poor prognosis for chronic SHP without antigen avoidance [20]. According to a national investigation of CHP conducted in Japan from 2000 to

2009, the median survival of 222 patients with CHP was 83 months. In this study, there were 33 cases (14.9%) of chronic SHP, and the median survival of patients with bird-related and home-related CHP did not differ significantly [22]. There are two important challenges in the treatment of chronic SHP. One is that the patient cannot easily remove the antigen from their home, and the other is that fibrosis may occur even after removal of the antigen.

Similar to other types of CHP, the effectiveness of corticosteroids for treating chronic SHP is low. The primary treatment is antigen avoidance by moving to another residence; however, if this is difficult, early cases without severe fibrosis can be treated with corticosteroid therapy.

In contrast, nintedanib is effective for treating progressive fibrosing interstitial lung disease (PF-ILD) [23]. As CHP is one of the main conditions leading to PF-ILD, nintedanib should be administered to patients with CHP if they show a gradual decline in pulmonary function.

References

1. Miyagawa T, Ochi T, Takahashi H. Hypersensitivity pneumonitis with antibodies to *Cryptococcus neoformans*. Clin Allergy. 1978;8:501–9.
2. Shimazu K, Ando M, Sakata T, et al. Hypersensitivity pneumonitis induced by *Trichosporon cutaneum*. Am Rev Respir Dis. 1984;130:407–11.
3. Yoshida K, Ando M, Sakata T, et al. Environmental mycological studies on the causative agent of summer-type hypersensitivity pneumonitis. J Allergy Clin Immunol. 1988;81:475–83.
4. Soda K, Ando M, Shimazu K, et al. Different classes of antibody activities to *Trichosporon cutaneum* antigen in summer-type hypersensitivity pneumonitis by enzyme-linked immunosorbent assay. Am Rev Respir Dis. 1986;133:83–7.
5. Ando M, Sakata T, Yoshida K, et al. Serotype-related antigen of *Trichosporon cutaneum* in the induction of summer-type hypersensitivity pneumonitis: correlation between serotype of inhalation challenge-positive antigen and that of the isolates from patients' homes. J Allergy Clin Immunol. 1990;85:36–44.
6. Ando M, Arima K, Yoneda R, et al. Japanese summer-type hypersensitivity pneumonitis. Geographic distribution, home environment, and clinical characteristics of 621 cases. Am Rev Respir Dis. 1991;144:765–9.
7. Sugita T, Ikeda R, Nishikawa A. Analysis of *Trichosporon* isolates obtained from the houses of patients with summer-type hypersensitivity pneumonitis. J Clin Microbiol. 2004;42:5467–71.
8. Unoura K, Miyazaki Y, Sumi Y, et al. Identification of fungal DNA in BALF from patients with home-related hypersensitivity pneumonitis. Respir Med. 2011;105:1696–703.
9. Asai N, Kaneko N, Ohkuni Y, Aoshima M, Kawamura Y. Familial summer-type hypersensitivity pneumonitis: a review of 25 families and 50 cases in Japan. Intern Med. 2016;55(3):279–83.
10. Ando M, Suga M, Nishiura Y, et al. Summer-type hypersensitivity pneumonitis. Intern Med. 1995;34:707–12.
11. Yoo CG, Kim YW, Han SK, et al. Summer-type hypersensitivity pneumonitis outside Japan: a case report and the state of the art. Respirology. 1997;2:75–7.
12. Okamoto T, Fujii M, Furusawa H, et al. The usefulness of KL-6 and SP-D for the diagnosis and management of chronic hypersensitivity pneumonitis. Respir Med. 2015;109:1576–81.
13. Ando M, Konishi K, Yoneda R, et al. Difference in the phenotypes of bronchoalveolar lavage lymphocytes in patients with summer-type hypersensitivity pneumonitis, farmer's lung, ven-

tilation pneumonitis, and bird fancier's lung: report of a nationwide epidemiologic study in Japan. J Allergy Clin Immunol. 1991;87:1002–9.

14. Raghu G, Remy-Jardin M, Ryerson CJ, et al. Diagnosis of hypersensitivity pneumonitis in adults. An official ATS/JRS/ALAT clinical practice guideline. Am J Respir Crit Care Med. 2020;202:e36–69.
15. Fernández Pérez ER, Travis WD, Lynch DA, et al. Diagnosis and evaluation of hypersensitivity pneumonitis: CHEST guideline and expert panel report. Chest. 2021;160:e97–e159.
16. Yoshida K, Ando M, Sakata T, et al. Prevention of summer-type hypersensitivity pneumonitis: effect of elimination of *Trichosporon cutaneum* from the patients' homes. Arch Environ Health. 1989;44:317–22.
17. Yoshizawa Y, Ohtani Y, Hayakawa H, et al. Chronic hypersensitivity pneumonitis in Japan: a nationwide epidemiologic survey. J Allergy Clin Immunol. 1999;103:315–20.
18. Onishi Y, Kawamura T, Higashino T, et al. Clinical features of chronic summer-type hypersensitivity pneumonitis and proposition of diagnostic criteria. Respir Investig. 2020;58:59–67.
19. Tsutsui T, Miyazaki Y, Okamoto T, et al. Antigen avoidance tests for diagnosis of chronic hypersensitivity pneumonitis. Respir Investig. 2015;53:217–24.
20. Inase N, Ohtani Y, Usui Y, et al. Chronic summer-type hypersensitivity pneumonitis: clinical similarities to idiopathic pulmonary fibrosis. Sarcoidosis Vasc Diffuse Lung Dis. 2007;24:141–7.
21. Ohtani Y, Ochi J, Mitaka K, et al. Chronic summer-type hypersensitivity pneumonitis initially misdiagnosed as idiopathic interstitial pneumonia. Intern Med. 2008;47:857–62.
22. Okamoto T, Miyazaki Y, Ogura T, et al. Nationwide epidemiological survey of chronic hypersensitivity pneumonitis in Japan. Respir Investig. 2013;51:191–9.
23. Flaherty KR, Wells AU, Cottin V, et al. Nintedanib in progressive fibrosing interstitial lung diseases. N Engl J Med. 2019;381:1718–27.

Chapter 14
Bird-Related Hypersensitivity Pneumonitis

What Is Bird-Related Hypersensitivity Pneumonitis?

Tomoya Tateishi

1 Introduction

In the 1960s, cases of hypersensitivity pneumonitis were documented among pigeon and parrot breeders, leading to the adoption of the terms "bird breeder's lung" or "bird fancier's lung (BFL) [1, 2]." This condition is a specific manifestation of hypersensitivity pneumonitis, a broader category of lung disease. BFL is often cited as a significant cause of hypersensitivity pneumonitis, alongside other forms such as summer-type hypersensitivity pneumonitis and farmer's lung [3]. In the United States and Europe, BFL represents the predominant antigenic cause of hypersensitivity pneumonitis, accounting for 34–67% of cases [4, 5]. Conversely, in Japan, the most frequently identified antigen in hypersensitivity pneumonitis is *Trichosporon asahii* [6, 7]. Epidemiological studies in Japan indicate that, while *Trichosporon asahii* is the most common antigen, BFL is the second most prevalent and the leading antigenic cause of fibrotic hypersensitivity pneumonitis [8]. This makes it the most common cause of fibrotic hypersensitivity pneumonitis in Japan.

In Japan, the initial report of the disease emerged in the 1970s among budgerigar breeders, initially termed as a bird-feeding-related illness. Since then, the number of cases has risen, leading to its recognition as a prevalent condition. Subsequent findings revealed that the disease could also be triggered by avian antigens in domestic settings, such as those found in feather duvets. Consequently, the term "bird-related hypersensitivity pneumonitis (BRHP)" is now deemed more accurate and encompassing than the earlier used "BFL."

T. Tateishi (✉)
Department of Respiratory Medicine, Institute of Science Tokyo, Tokyo, Japan
e-mail: tateishi.pulm@tmd.ac.jp

Y. Miyazaki (ed.), *Hypersensitivity Pneumonitis*, Respiratory Disease Series: Diagnostic Tools and Disease Managements,
https://doi.org/10.1007/978-981-96-7983-6_14

2 Causative Antigen

Most birds involved in bird breeding, particularly in the context of pigeon racing, are pigeons and doves. Due to their robust homing instincts, doves are primarily used in pigeon racing, a well-established pastime in Europe and North America. Since the 1970s, pigeon racing has also gained popularity in Japan and China, predominantly among middle-aged and older individuals, as a recreational hobby.

Exposure to avian antigens outside of breeding contexts is prevalent in urban areas. Due to the scarcity of natural predators, doves often nest in elevated locations such as apartment balconies and attics, inadvertently elevating the concentration of avian antigens in residential settings. Starlings are also commonly observed in urban environments [5]. While the bird species vary across different countries and regions, bird antigens are generally considered cross-specific, indicating that nearly all bird species can potentially be causative antigens [9].

The primary antigens in this context are from birds within the order Psittaciformes, including budgerigars, cockatiels, parrots, parakeets, and canaries. Additionally, the disease is believed to be associated with the domestication of poultry such as chickens, turkeys, geese, and ducks.

In addition to direct exposure to birds, including activities like bird breeding, cases of the disease have been linked to indirect sources such as the use of poultry manure as fertilizer and products containing down, like down quilts and jackets.

It is estimated that fewer than 10% of individuals exposed to avian antigens develop BRHP. This condition does not invariably occur, even among those living in the same environment as the antigens. The exact cause associated with developing BRHP is unknown, although it is thought to be influenced by various factors such as gender, smoking status, genetic predisposition, and the amount of exposure. Consequently, the incidence of BRHP among those exposed to avian antigens is believed to be below 10% [10].

3 Antigen

It is hypothesized that organic substances from the intestinal tract and blood contribute to the antigenic components in bird droppings and feathers. Previously identified antigens included immunoglobulin A (IgA), immunoglobulin G (IgG), and mucins originating from the intestinal tract. However, recent studies have brought attention to pigeon immunoglobulin-lambda-like polypeptide-1 (IGLL-1), commonly found in pigeon feces and serum, as a potential causative antigen for the disease [9, 11]. The initial report suggested IGLL-1 as a causative antigen, and subsequent findings indicate that pigeon IGLL-1, also present in the feces of several bird species, may be a causative antigen in birds other than pigeons.

4 Clinical Features

The clinical progression of nonfibrotic BRHP, including acute and subacute forms, is comparable to that caused by other antigens. However, BRHP is distinct in its high incidence of progressing to fibrotic hypersensitivity pneumonitis [12, 13]. Notably, in patients initially presenting with acute symptoms and diagnosed with nonfibrotic hypersensitivity pneumonitis, the detection of residual ground-glass or infiltrative opacities on CT scans years later can raise suspicions regarding the progression to fibrotic hypersensitivity pneumonitis.

The clinical course of fibrotic BRHP can be categorized into two types: the recurrent type, characterized by progressive fibrosis accompanying recurrent symptoms such as low-grade fever and dyspnea, and the insidious type, where the disease is identified in an advanced state of dyspnea with minimal prior symptoms [12]. The subclinical form often includes cases diagnosed with significant interstitial changes at presentation. In the recurrent type, an increase in interstitial changes is also observed over several years. The insidious type typically presents in a state of advanced respiratory distress.

5 Immunological Test

5.1 Serum-Specific Antibodies

Previously, serum bird-associated antibodies were only measurable in specialized laboratories, but since 2020, bird-specific IgG can be quantified using the ImmunoCAP® method [14]. This method is highly sensitive for detecting causative antigens in the patients with nonfibrotic hypersensitivity pneumonia. In cases of fibrotic hypersensitivity pneumonia, the sensitivity and specificity of antibodies to pigeons are approximately 33% and 86%, respectively, which are somewhat lower than those for nonfibrotic forms. However, combining antibodies to pigeons and parrots improves the diagnostic utility, yielding a relatively good sensitivity of 61% and specificity of 75%. This makes it a useful tool for screening and diagnosis. Conversely, it is important to note that bird-associated antibodies are detected in over 80% of healthy individuals who keep birds in one cohort, indicating sensitization rather than disease [15].

5.2 Lymphocyte Stimulation Test

The lymphocyte stimulation test serves as an adjunct to the serum-specific antibody test in evaluating chronic avian hypersensitivity pneumonia. In this test, pigeon serum or pigeon feces extract is introduced to lymphocytes isolated from peripheral blood. The rate of lymphocyte proliferation following this exposure is then measured. It is important to note that the lymphocyte stimulation test alone does not offer high sensitivity for chronic bird-related hypersensitivity pneumonia, as it demonstrates a sensitivity of 46% and a specificity of 91% [16]. Therefore, a comprehensive diagnosis should be made in conjunction with other tests.

5.3 *Inhalation Provocation Test*

One key diagnostic criterion for hypersensitivity pneumonitis is the reproducibility of symptoms upon exposure to the suspected antigen. To evaluate this, inhalation challenge tests are employed. Specifically, for avian-associated hypersensitivity pneumonitis, inhalation challenge tests have been conducted using pigeon feces extract, pigeon serum, and pigeon eggs [17, 18]. These tests aim to identify the specific antigen triggering hypersensitivity pneumonitis. However, despite their utility in antigen identification, the American College of Chest Physicians (ACCP) guidelines do not actively recommend these tests for routine diagnosis of hypersensitivity pneumonitis, due to potential risks and limitations associated with their use [19].

6 Case 1

A female office worker in her 40 s presented at the Interstitial Lung Disease (ILD) clinic with complaints of cough and mild fever. She had been keeping ornamental pigeons at her home for 2 years. Initially, she was diagnosed with an upper respiratory tract infection at a local clinic, but her symptoms persisted. Two weeks later, she experienced mMRC grade 2 dyspnea upon exertion. High-resolution computed tomography (HRCT) revealed diffuse granular shadows, raising suspicions of non-fibrotic hypersensitivity pneumonitis (Fig. 14.1a). Bronchoalveolar lavage fluid analysis showed a markedly elevated lymphocyte ratio of 90%. Transbronchial lung biopsy revealed lymphocytic interstitial pneumonitis and granulomas. Testing for bird-specific IgG antibodies returned positive results. The patient was admitted for management, which included education on antigen avoidance, and was subsequently discharged. She ceased pigeon rearing, and since then, has had no recurrence of symptoms.

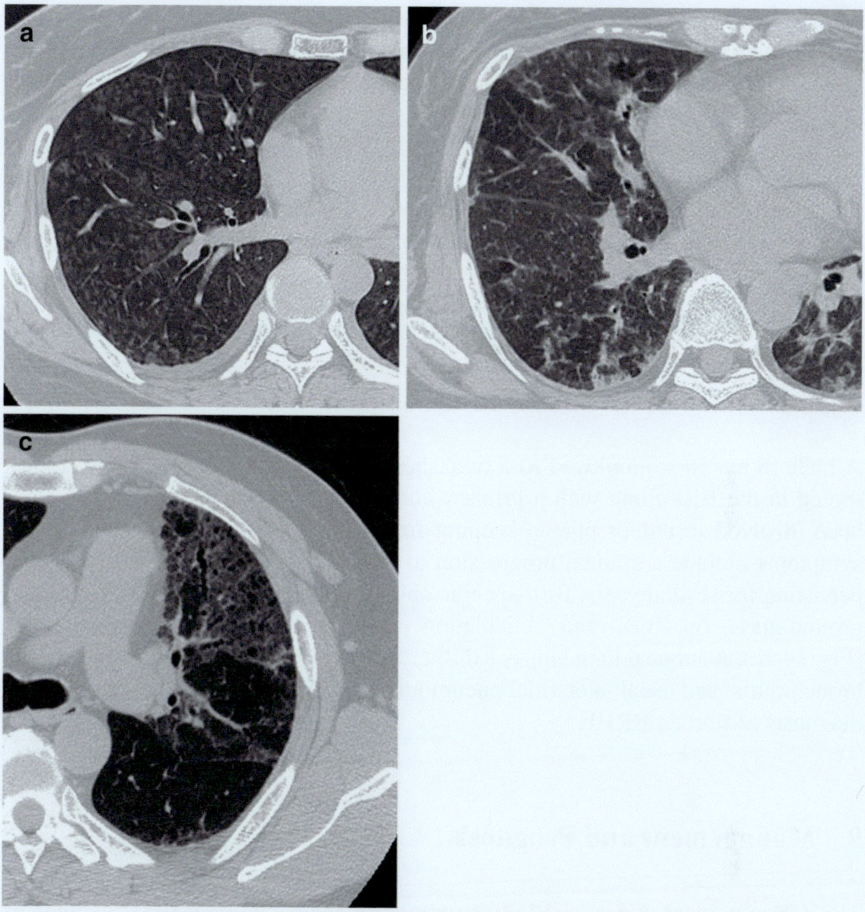

Fig. 14.1 (**a**) High-resolution CT (HRCT) findings of the patient with nonfibrotic bird-related hypersensitivity pneumonitis (BRHP). (**b**) HRCT findings of the patient with recurrent type of fibrotic BRHP. (**c**) HRCT findings of the patient with insidious type of fibrotic BRHP

7 Case 2

A female homemaker in her 60 s, who has never smoked, experienced recurrent episodes of cough, fever, and mMRC grade 2 dyspnea upon exertion over the past 5 years. There is no exposure to mold antigens at home; however, there is a pigeon coop located in a park directly in front of the house, housing approximately 300 pigeons. HRCT revealed diffuse interstitial shadows with a mosaic pattern and a three-density pattern (Fig. 14.1b) [20]. A surgical lung biopsy demonstrated airway-centered fibrosis, along with lymphocytic interstitial pneumonitis and granulomas involving epithelial cells. Antigen avoidance for 2 weeks resulted in improved respiratory function and a positive antigen avoidance test result [21–23]. Following a multidisciplinary discussion, she was diagnosed with fibrotic hypersensitivity pneumonitis, characterized by diminishing recurrent symptoms. For effective antigen avoidance, she decided to move out of her house.

8 Case 3

A male in his 50 s, employed as a bookshop manager and a current smoker, presented to the ILD clinic with a primary complaint of exertional dyspnea. He has been involved in indoor pigeon keeping for magic tricks for over 30 years. His symptoms include a gradual progression to mMRC grade 2 dyspnea on exertion, persisting for several years. Bird-specific antibodies were positive. HRCT revealed ground-glass opacities and reticulation along the bronchovascular bundles (Fig. 14.1c). A surgical lung biopsy exhibited airway-centered fibrosis, lymphocytic bronchiolitis, and usual interstitial pneumonia (UIP) patterns. A MDD concluded a diagnosis of fibrotic BRHP.

9 Management and Prognosis

The cornerstone of hypersensitivity pneumonitis management is the avoidance of the triggering antigen (refer to Chap. 11) [24]. However, it is crucial to acknowledge that antigen avoidance alone may be insufficient in advanced stages of the disease. In cases where hypersensitivity pneumonitis progresses despite avoidance of the causative antigen, pharmacotherapy should be considered (refer to Chap. 12) [25]. This is particularly pertinent in BRHP, where there is a heightened risk of developing fibrotic hypersensitivity pneumonitis. The risk of fibrosis in BRHP is notably higher compared to hypersensitivity pneumonitis induced by other antigens. Given the diverse range of antigens implicated in BRHP, it is crucial to periodically assess whether patients are effectively avoiding antigen exposure. This approach is essential to prevent the progression of fibrosis due to unrecognized antigen exposure.

The prognosis for fibrotic BRHP shows considerable variability, as evidenced by 5-year survival rates ranging from 30% to 60% [26, 27]. Data on antigen-limited fibrotic hypersensitivity pneumonitis are limited, with few reports addressing multiple cases. In contrast, the 5-year survival rate for fibrotic hypersensitivity pneumonitis in general is estimated to be between 60% and 70% [28].

10 Case 4

A female homemaker in her 70 s presented to the ILD clinic with a history of cough, sputum production, and exertional dyspnea persisting for several years. She reported a 20-year history of indoor canary keeping. She was diagnosed with nonfibrotic BRHP and advised to cease bird keeping and eliminate bird antigens from her environment. Six years later, she experienced a gradual exacerbation of dyspnea upon exertion and returned for evaluation. It was discovered that the patient had resumed using down quilts and down jackets a few years prior. She was under the misconception that discontinuing bird rearing alone would prevent a recurrence of her BRHP.

11 Conclusion

Bird-related hypersensitivity pneumonitis (BRHP) frequently progresses to a fibrotic stage and clinically resembles idiopathic interstitial pneumonias in its manifestations. Among various types of hypersensitivity pneumonitis, differentiating BRHP from idiopathic interstitial pneumonia is crucial. Accurate identification of the causative antigen can potentially improve prognosis. Therefore, in the management of diffuse lung diseases, clinicians should diligently assess exposure to avian antigens through patient interviews.

References

1. Reed CE, Barbee RA. Pigeon-breeders' lung: a newly observed interstitial pulmonary disease. JAMA. 1965;193:261–5.
2. Hargreave FE, Pepys J, Longbottom JL, Wraith DG. Bird breeder's (fancier's) lung. Proc R Soc Med. 1966;59(10):1008.
3. Chan AL, Juarez MM, Leslie KO, Ismail HA, Albertson TE. Bird fancier's lung: a state-of-the-art review. Clin Rev Allergy Immunol. 2012;43(1–2):69–83.
4. Hanak V, Golbin JM, Ryu JH. Causes and presenting features in 85 consecutive patients with hypersensitivity pneumonitis. Mayo Clin Proc. 2007;82(7):812–6.
5. Borderías L, Morell F, Vera J, Briz H, Muñoz X, Cruz MJ. Starling-induced hypersensitivity pneumonitis: minimal but persistent antigen exposure. Arch Bronconeumol. 2010;46(11):607–9.
6. Yoshizawa Y, Ohtani Y, Hayakawa H, Sato A, Suga M, Ando M. Chronic hypersensitivity pneumonitis in Japan: a nationwide epidemiologic survey. J Allergy Clin Immunol. 1999;103(2):315–20.
7. Okamoto T, Miyazaki Y, Ogura T, Chida K, Kohno N, Kohno S, et al. A nationwide epidemiological survey of chronic hypersensitivity pneumonitis in Japan. Respir Investig. 2013;51(3):191–9.
8. Lacasse Y, Selman M, Costabel U, Dalphin J-C, Morell F, Erkinjuntti-Pekkanen R, et al. Classification of hypersensitivity pneumonitis. Int Arch Allergy Immunol. 2009;149(2):161–6.
9. Shirai T, Furusawa H, Furukawa A, Ishige Y, Uchida K, Miyazaki Y, et al. Protein antigen of bird-related hypersensitivity pneumonitis in pigeon serum and dropping. Respir Res. 2017;18(1):65.

10. Fink JN, Schlueter DP, Sosman AJ, Unger GF, Barboriak JJ, Rimm AA, et al. Clinical survey of pigeon breeders. Chest. 1972;62(3):277–81.
11. Rouzet A, Reboux G, Dalphin J-C, Gondouin A, De Vuyst P, Balliau T, et al. An immunoproteomic approach revealed antigenic proteins enhancing serodiagnosis performance of bird fancier's lung. J Immunol Methods. 2017;450:58–65.
12. Ohtani Y, Saiki S, Sumi Y, Inase N, Miyake S, Costabel U, et al. Clinical features of recurrent and insidious chronic bird fancier's lung. Ann Allergy Asthma Immunol. 2003;90(6):604–10.
13. Tateishi T, Ohtani Y, Takemura T, Akashi T, Miyazaki Y, Inase N, et al. Serial high-resolution computed tomography findings of acute and chronic hypersensitivity pneumonitis induced by avian antigen. J Comput Assist Tomogr. 2011;35(2):272–9.
14. Shirai T, Tanino Y, Nikaido T, Takaku Y, Hashimoto S, Taguchi Y, et al. Screening and diagnosis of acute and chronic bird-related hypersensitivity pneumonitis by serum IgG and IgA antibodies to bird antigens with ImmunoCAP(R). Allergol Int. 2020;
15. Morell F, Roger À, Reyes L, Cruz MJ, Murio C, Muñoz X. Bird fancier's lung: a series of 86 patients. Medicine (Baltimore). 2008;87(2):110–30.
16. Suhara K, Miyazaki Y, Okamoto T, Yasui M, Tsuchiya K, Inase N. Utility of immunological tests for bird-related hypersensitivity pneumonitis. Respir Investig. 2015;53(1):13–21.
17. Ishizuka M, Miyazaki Y, Tateishi T, Tsutsui T, Tsuchiya K, Inase N. Validation of inhalation provocation test in chronic bird-related hypersensitivity pneumonitis and new prediction score. Ann Am Thorac Soc. 2015;12(2):167–73.
18. Okuda R, Takemura T, Mikami Y, Hagiwara E, Iwasawa T, Baba T, et al. Inhalation challenge test using pigeon eggs for chronic hypersensitivity pneumonitis. Clin Exp Allergy. 2020;50(12):1381–90.
19. Fernández Pérez ER, Travis WD, Lynch DA, Brown KK, Johannson KA, Selman M, et al. Executive summary diagnosis and evaluation of hypersensitivity pneumonitis. Chest. 2021;160:e97.
20. Barnett J, Molyneaux PL, Rawal B, Abdullah R, Hare SS, Vancheeswaran R, et al. Variable utility of mosaic attenuation to distinguish fibrotic hypersensitivity pneumonitis from idiopathic pulmonary fibrosis. Eur Respir J. 2019;54(1):1900531.
21. Tsutsui T, Miyazaki Y, Okamoto T, Tateishi T, Furusawa H, Tsuchiya K, et al. Antigen avoidance tests for diagnosis of chronic hypersensitivity pneumonitis. Respir Investig. 2015;53(5):217–24.
22. Okuda R, Takemura T, Iwasawa T, Kaburaki S, Baba T, Hagiwara E, et al. Impact of antigen avoidance test for fibrotic hypersensitivity pneumonitis in stable phase. Allergy, Asthma Clin Immunol. 2022;18(1):104.
23. Hanzawa S, Tateishi T, Ishizuka M, Inoue Y, Honda T, Kawahara T, et al. Changes in serum KL-6 levels during short-term strict antigen avoidance are associated with the prognosis of patients with fibrotic hypersensitivity pneumonitis caused by avian antigens. Respir Investig. 2020;58(6):457–64.
24. Tsutsui T, Miyazaki Y, Kuramochi J, Uchida K, Eishi Y, Inase N. The amount of avian antigen in household dust predicts the prognosis of chronic bird-related hypersensitivity pneumonitis. Ann Am Thorac Soc. 2015;12(7):1013–21.
25. De Sadeleer LJ, Hermans F, De Dycker E, Yserbyt J, Verschakelen JA, Verbeken EK, et al. Effects of corticosteroid treatment and antigen avoidance in a large hypersensitivity pneumonitis Cohort: a single-centre Cohort study. J Clin Med. 2019;8(1):14.
26. Pérez-Padilla R, Salas J, Chapela R, Sánchez M, Carrillo G, Pérez R, et al. Mortality in Mexican patients with chronic pigeon breeder's lung compared with those with usual interstitial pneumonia. Am Rev Respir Dis. 1993;148(1):49–53.
27. Ohtani Y, Saiki S, Kitaichi M, Usui Y, Inase N, Costabel U, et al. Chronic bird fancier's lung: histopathological and clinical correlation. An application of the 2002 ATS/ERS consensus classification of the idiopathic interstitial pneumonias. Thorax. 2005;60(8):665–71.
28. Alberti ML, Malet Ruiz JM, Fernández ME, Fassola L, Caro F, Roldán IB, et al. Comparative survival analysis between idiopathic pulmonary fibrosis and chronic hypersensitivity pneumonitis. Pulmonology. 2020;26(1):3–9.

Chapter 15
Humidifier's Lung

What Is Humidifier's Lungs?

Susumu Sakamoto

Abbreviations

BALF	Bronchoalveolar lavage fluid
BNP	Brain natriuretic peptide
CRP	C-reactive protein
FEV1	Forced expiratory volume in 1 second
KL-6	Krebs von der Lungen-6
LDH	Lactate dehydrogenase
SP-A	Surfactant protein A
SP-D	Surfactant protein D
VC	Vital capacity
%DLCO	Carbon-monoxide-diffusing capacity % of predicted value
%VC	Vital capacity % of predicted value

1 Introduction

Hypersensitivity pneumonitis (HP) is caused by continuous inhalation of various antigens. The diagnosis of HP requires identification of antigens; hence, challenge tests are useful. Symptoms improve when patients avoid antigen exposure, but some patients need and benefit from corticosteroid (CS) treatment. HP is classified in relation to the causative antigen as summer-type HP, humidifier lung, bird breeders' lung, hot-tub lung, and farmers' lung [1]. Humid weather conditions in Japan, in addition to traditional wooden houses, increase exposure to *Trichosporon asahii*. This has led to reports of a high incidence of summer-type HP in Japan—greater than 70%—and its characteristics are thus well understood [2, 3]. However, few studies have assessed humidifier lung.

S. Sakamoto (✉)
Division of Respiratory Medicine, Toho University Omori Medical Center, Tokyo, Japan

Y. Miyazaki (ed.), *Hypersensitivity Pneumonitis*, Respiratory Disease Series: Diagnostic Tools and Disease Managements,
https://doi.org/10.1007/978-981-96-7983-6_15

The use of ultrasonic humidifiers is common in Japan, specifically to prevent dry indoor environments during winter. Humidifier lung, a type of home environmental HP, is also known as "humidifier fever" or "Monday morning sickness". The term is also used to describe HP caused by inhalational exposure to contaminated ventilation units. The first report of HP associated with a contaminated humidifier was published in 1970. Pestalozzi described it as humidifier fever in 1959, and Banaszak et al. reported it as HP in 1970 [4]. This condition is classified as one of the several types of HP, and the pathogenesis is presumed to involve endotoxin in addition to type III and IV allergic reactions [1–3].

Contaminated ultrasonic humidifiers directly disperse causative antigens in 0.5–3-μm droplets that easily reach distal airway spaces. Water in poorly cleaned ultrasonic humidifiers is easily contaminated with microorganisms such as bacteria, fungi, and nontuberculous mycobacteria, including endotoxins [4–12].

Thermophilic actinomycetes have been isolated from humidifier water, and the precipitating antibodies have been implicated as a cause of humidifier lung. However, several studies found that in some cases, humidifier lung was not caused by these organisms; thus, humidifier lung might be caused by multiple antigens. Generally, prolonged exposure to a contaminating fungal or bacterial antigen and/or endotoxin results in immune sensitization and causes immune-mediated lung injury in susceptible individuals [4–12].

The criteria for diagnosing this rare condition are not standardized, and the clinical, laboratory, and chest CT features of humidifier lung are not well documented. We hypothesize that the mechanism underlying humidifier lung differs from that of common summer-type HP. However, few studies have reported on the comprehensive evaluation of humidifier lung [11].

In this chapter, we focus on the results of a comparison of clinical, laboratory, CT findings, and pathological features of humidifier lung with those of summer-type HP, the most common HP in Japan that we have previously reported [13].

2 Etiology

Humidifier lung is caused by repeated inhalation of humidifier water contaminated with bacteria, fungi, acidophiles, and endotoxins, and is triggered by further inhalation of contaminated water. The pathogenesis of humidifier lung and other types of HP is considered to be similar. Type III and type IV hypersensitivity reactions to bacteria and/or fungal antigens are involved; however, previous studies found that the type IV hypersensitivity reaction was more significant [1, 14].

The causative antigens include bacteria such as *Thermophilic actinomycetes, Thermoactinomyces vulgaris, Thermoactinomyces candidus, Flavobacterium meningosepticum, Candida albicans, Cephalosporium acremonium, Trichoderma viride, Aspergillus fumigatus,* and other fungi. Amoeba such as *Naegleria gruberi* has been reported as causative antigens also. Of these reports, those cases with suggested involvement of thermophilic microorganisms involved heated humidifiers, but most household humidifiers used in Japan are of the ultrasonic type, and there have been few reports on thermophilic microorganisms. Persons with humidifier lung sometimes have specific detectable immune-mediated reactions, such as precipitating antibodies and proliferation of lymphocytes against humidifier water.

There have been reports of cases involving Gram-negative rods with elevated endotoxin levels in humidifier water and blood, suggesting that endotoxin may be involved in the pathogenesis of fever and leukocytosis [1–3, 15–18].

Summer-type HP seems to be caused by continuous exposure to a small amount of fungal antigens. In contrast, patients with humidifier lung may develop pulmonary and systemic symptoms after direct exposure to a large amount of highly antigenic particles, such as bacteria and fungi and/or endotoxins, while using humidifiers with highly polluted water. The pathophysiology of humidifier lung may thus encompass not only hypersensitivity reactions such as HP but also endotoxin-induced lung injury. Gram-negative bacteria and their associated endotoxins may be involved in the pathogenesis of humidifier lung, as humidifier water contains high levels of endotoxins [15–18]. Endotoxins are an extremely potent agent of lung injury, and endotoxin inhalation can cause pulmonary and systemic symptoms by inducing inflammatory cytokines such as interleukin-1 and tumor necrosis factor-alpha, in addition to neutrophilia as well as lymphocytosis in BALF and peripheral blood [19, 20]. Recent studies have described considerable interindividual variability in endotoxin responsiveness. This variability is based on polymorphisms in genes encoding proinflammatory cytokines, LPS receptor CD14 in humans, and Toll-like receptors. Variability in endotoxin sensitivity may thus contribute to differences in clinical and radiological features among patients with humidifier lung [21–25].

3 Diagnosis of Humidifier Lung

The criteria for diagnosing this rare condition have not been standardized; however, the ATS/JRS/ALAT Guidelines for the Diagnosis of Hypersensitivity Pneumonitis (GL for HP) were published in 2020 [26] followed by the CHEST Guidelines for the Diagnosis and Evaluation of Hypersensitivity Pneumonitis [27] in 2021. Few studies have comprehensively evaluated the utility of these guidelines for diagnosing humidifier lung. Therefore, examining the level of diagnostic confidence for humidifier lung using these guidelines for HP is requisite.

In our previous study, humidifier lung was diagnosed from clinical and radiological findings by using a previously reported method [11] and the following criteria: (1) persisting respiratory symptoms (such as cough, sputum, and dyspnea) for longer than 1 week; (2) bilateral ground-glass opacity or consolidation on chest CT; (3) history of home ultrasonic humidifier use; (4) positive result on a provocation test; (5) bronchoalveolar lavage fluid (BALF) findings or histopathological findings consistent with HP; and (6) improved symptoms, laboratory findings, and chest high-resolution CT (HRCT) images after cessation of home ultrasonic humidifier use. Humidifier lung was diagnosed based on the presence of criteria 1, 2, 3, 4, and 5; criteria 1, 2, 3, 5, and 6; criteria 1, 2, 3, and 4; or criteria 1, 2, 3, and 6 (probable).

4 Provocation Testing

Presently, there is no established method for performing provocation tests for humidifier lung. The following protocol is applied for provocation testing at our institution. The humidifier is operated in a hospital room measuring approximately 20 m^2, with all windows and doors closed. The patient's humidifier is placed at the bedside, and they are exposed to humidifier mist for 2 h. If they develop symptoms during exposure, the challenge test is stopped. Symptoms and vital signs are then observed over the next 24 h. Information is collected on body temperature, total and differential white blood cell (WBC) count, serum C-reactive protein (CRP), lactate dehydrogenase (LDH), Krebs von den Lungen 6 (KL-6), surfactant protein-A (SP-A), surfactant protein-D (SP-D) levels, arterial blood gas analysis, pulmonary function test results, and HRCT image findings. Patients who develop symptoms from inhaling ultrasonic humidifier mist are classified as having a positive result. All patients undergoing the test give their written informed consent first. In most cases, humidifier avoidance or removal would result in resolution of both respiratory symptoms and abnormalities in blood test results. A few patients have developed acute respiratory failure needing corticosteroid treatment after the provocation test. Hence, performing provocation tests requires that facilities have appropriate equipment and medications to adequately manage acute respiratory failure.

5 Patient Characteristics

In our study, most patients with humidifier lung first visited the hospital in winter. As our previously reported findings suggest, the duration of symptoms ranged from 1 to 9 weeks (median, 2 weeks). Most of the patients had home ultrasonic humidifiers and used tap water in the humidifiers. The duration of humidifier use ranged from 1 to 4 months during the period of September through March [15].

As with summer HP, subacute to acute disease, with dyspnea, cough, and fever, was most common. Although other family members were exposed to the humidifiers, none developed humidifier lung. Fine crackles were the most prominent physical finding. In mild cases, these symptoms improved within a relatively short period of time after avoiding the use of humidifiers [11, 12, 15]. Patients with humidifier lung often have episodes of recurrent pneumonia. They are occasionally admitted for a diagnosis of bacterial pneumonia with fever, cough, and chest radiograph abnormality. On hospitalization, they are treated with antibiotics and their condition improves. For some patients, however, their symptoms worsen, and their condition deteriorates shortly after discharge, leading to rehospitalization. Such episodes suggest a high index of suspicion for humidifier lung.

6 Laboratory Findings

Serum levels of CRP and LDH, in addition to WBC counts, were elevated in most patients. The WBC counts and serum CRP levels were higher for humidifier lung than for summer-type HP. Analysis of differential WBC cell counts showed that the lymphocyte fraction was lower for humidifier lung than for summer-type HP. The neutrophil fraction was higher for humidifier lung than for summer-type HP.

Unlike typical summer-type HP, serum KL-6 and SP-D levels were significantly lower in patients with humidifier lung than in those with summer-type HP. Shimoda et al. also examined these indicators and reported similar trends [28]. Serum KL-6 levels were not elevated during the clinical course in most patients with humidifier lung. Increases in serum KL-6 and SP-D are thought to be a hallmark of summer-type HP and farmers' lung [15, 28, 29]. However, serum SP-D level was elevated in almost all patients with humidifier lung. In summer-type HP, prolonged low-level antigen exposure leads to subacute or chronic disease and, ultimately, to type IV allergy. Chronic inflammation causes alveolar fibrosis due to lymphocyte infiltration, epithelioid granuloma formation, and fibroblast activation. As fibrosis insidiously progresses, serum levels of interstitial lung disease markers, such as KL-6 and SP-D, rise concurrently. In contrast, because a large amount of antigen is inhaled during a short period of time in humidifier lung, onset of symptoms occurred early and many did not develop pulmonary fibrosis. Thus, increases in serum KL-6 and SP-D levels were comparatively lower for humidifier lung than for summer-type HP.

7 Pulmonary Function Testing

Few reports have evaluated respiratory function in humidifier lung. In our previous study, two of 18 (11.1%) patients with humidifier lung had restrictive impairment of respiratory function. One of 18 (5.6%) patients developed obstructive impairment of respiratory function. The decrease in DLCO was significantly less severe for humidifier lung than for summer-type HP [15].

8 Chest Radiograph

Chest radiographs sometimes show bilateral faint ground-glass opacity or consolidation. If present, bilateral consolidation suggests the differential diagnoses of bacterial pneumonia, pulmonary edema, other interstitial lung diseases, and pulmonary hemorrhage. In practice, many cases of humidifier lung are inadvertently treated initially as bacterial pneumonia before specialist review by a pulmonologist.

9 HRCT Findings

The most common HRCT findings for humidifier lung were faint ground-glass opacity and mosaic attenuation (Fig. 15.1a and b). Poorly defined centrilobular micronodules were less common in humidifier lung than in summer-type HP (Fig. 15.1c and d). Some patients with humidifier lung had unusual findings, as compared with summer-type HP. Chest HRCT scans showed bilateral ground-glass opacity and/or consolidation, without centrilobular ground-glass micronodules, in humidifier lung. Other patients with humidifier lung had diffuse peribronchovascular or subpleural nonsegmental consolidation bilaterally, which is unusual for non-fibrotic HP. These forms of consolidation were more frequent in humidifier lung than in summer-type HP (Fig. 15.1b). Consolidation on chest HRCT might be attributable to strong inflammatory reactions, including lung injury due to exposure to high levels of antigen and/or endotoxin.

During follow-up, HRCT findings gradually improved with avoidance of humidifier exposure and were almost normal at the end of follow-up. Ground-glass opacity developed after provocation testing but improved with avoidance of humidifier exposure or after corticosteroid treatment.

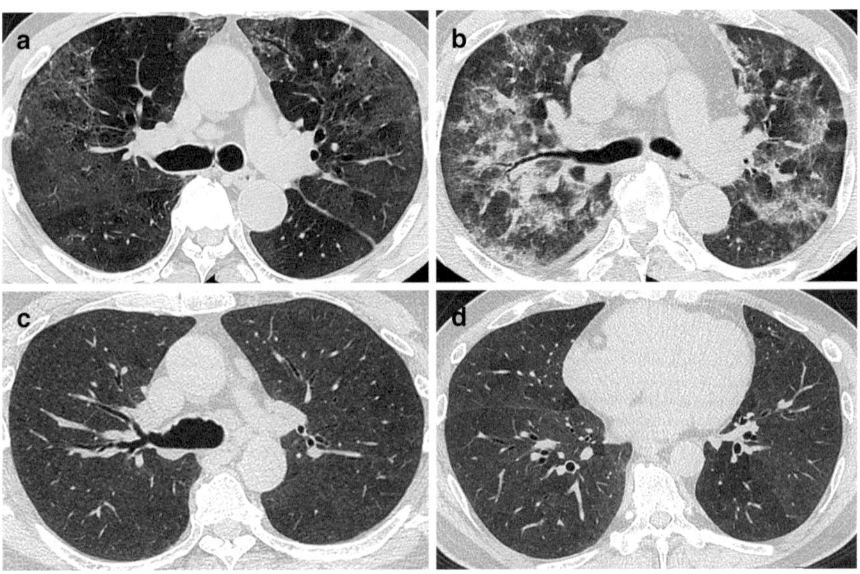

Fig. 15.1 Representative chest HRCT findings for humidifier lung. (**a**) Diffuse faint ground-glass opacity and mosaic attenuation, without poorly defined centrilobular micronodules. Diagnosis was made by provocation test. (**b**) Diffuse bilateral nonsegmental peribronchovascular consolidation, with intralobular septal thickening—an unusual finding for summer-type HP. Diagnosis was made by provocation test. (**c** and **d**). Representative chest HRCT scan for typical summer-type HP showing diffuse ground-glass opacity with poorly defined micronodules (**c**) and mosaic attenuation 3 (**d**)

Conversely, summer-type HP was generally associated with diffuse ground-glass opacity and poorly defined micronodules, predominantly in the middle to lower lung lobes [2, 3, 15, 28].

10 BALF Analysis

In our study, patients with humidifier lung had high total BALF cell counts, as did those with summer-type HP. Although there was no significant difference in total cell count, lymphocytosis was less for humidifier lung than for summer-type HP in BALF differential cell counts. Neutrophil fraction was greater for humidifier lung than for summer-type HP. Furthermore, the phenotypes of BAL lymphocytes differed significantly; CD4+ lymphocytes were predominant in humidifier lung, whereas CD8+ lymphocytes were predominant in summer-type HP. Thus, the CD4/CD8 ratio was significantly higher for humidifier lung than for summer-type HP.

Many studies have examined the surface phenotype of BAL lymphocytes in HP. Most HP patients exhibit an increase in BAL T lymphocytes, which are predominantly CD8+ lymphocytes, thus decreasing the CD4/CD8 ratio. However, CD4/CD8 ratio is higher in farmers' lung, which indicates that BAL lymphocyte phenotypes may depend on the type of HP [2, 3, 11, 30–32]. Few studies of humidifier lung have evaluated the phenotype of BAL lymphocytes [3, 11, 15, 28]. According to Suda et al., CD4/CD8 ratio was significantly higher for humidifier lung than for summer-type HP, which is consistent with our results [11]. Furthermore, the increase in the BALF neutrophil fraction was greater than that for summer-type HP. The reasons for these differences in WBC fractions and phenotypes of BAL lymphocytes in HP are unclear. As mentioned above, the nature or amount of inhaled causative antigens and endotoxins may explain these findings.

11 Pathological Findings

A few reports have examined the pathologic findings of humidifier lung in detail. In our study, examination of transbronchial lung biopsy specimens from 9 patients with humidifier lung revealed alveolar septal wall thickening with lymphocyte infiltration (alveolitis) in all patients (Fig. 15.2). Intra-alveolar organization was observed in 4 of the 9 patients. No patient had characteristics of epithelioid cell granuloma. Alveolitis and intra-alveolar macrophage infiltration were less severe than in summer-type HP [15].

Shimoda et al. also reported on pathologic findings in humidifier lung. They showed that there were no cases of epithelioid cell granuloma in humidifier lung [28].

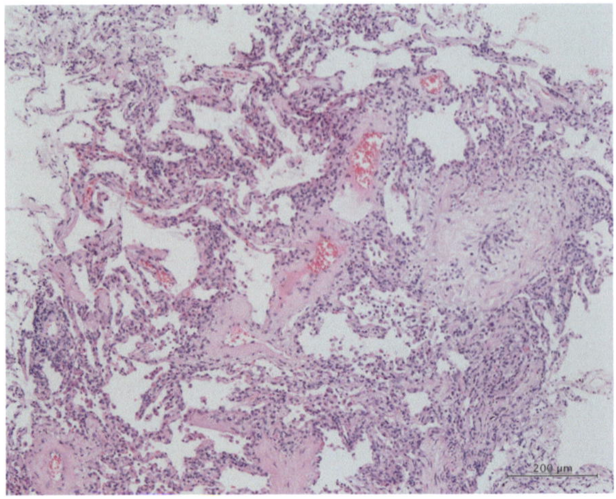

Fig. 15.2 Histopathological findings of transbronchial lung biopsy specimen showing diffuse alveolitis with lymphocyte infiltration and intra-alveolar organization (hematoxylin and eosin; scale bar 200 μm)

12 Treatments and Outcomes

Humidifier lung can readily resolve with antigen avoidance, and mild cases quickly improve with humidifier avoidance or removal. In most patients, we found that symptoms and blood test results and HRCT findings improved after humidifier avoidance and never recurred. Prednisolone was given at an initial dose of 0.5 mg/kg, and tapered off gradually. In our study, of all patients with humidifier lung, only about 30% needed corticosteroid treatment. Therefore, corticosteroid use was less frequent, and duration was shorter for humidifier lung than summer-type HP. In contrast, some patients were in severe respiratory failure at diagnosis. These patients received methylprednisolone pulse therapy (1000 mg/day over 3 days) as management of severe respiratory failure [15]. Even in severe cases, the response to therapeutic corticosteroids is relatively favorable, and most of the cases resolve without progressing to lung fibrosis. Although no detailed epidemiologic data exist, our study suggests that the prognosis is favorable provided diagnosis is accurate, and appropriate antigen avoidance and treatment are instituted.

13 Conclusion

The clinical and radiologic findings of humidifier lung differed from those of summer-type HP. Humidifier lung is sometimes difficult to diagnose as HP. Rapid diagnosis can be achieved by obtaining a detailed environmental history. The current ATS/JRS/ALAT diagnostic guidelines for hypersensitivity pneumonitis need to be validated for the diagnosis of humidifier lung and if diagnosis is still difficult to make, a unique set of criteria is beneficial for the definitive diagnosis of humidifier lung. It is necessary to accumulate more cases in the future to clarify the clinical features of humidifier lung, elucidate the pathogenesis, and develop diagnostic criteria specific to humidifier lung.

Acknowledgments We thank Florence Ene, MD, PhD, for medical English language editing of this chapter.

Funding/Support Statement None

Declaration of Competing Interest We declare that we have no conflict of interest.

References

1. Patel AM, Ryu JH, Reed CE. Hypersensitivity pneumonitis: current concepts and future questions. J Allergy Clin Immunol. 2001;108:661–70. https://doi.org/10.1067/mai.2001.119570.
2. Ando M, Suga M, Kohrogi H. A new look at hypersensitivity pneumonitis. Curr Opin Pulm Med. 1999;5:299–304. https://doi.org/10.1097/00063198-199909000-00006.
3. Ando M, Konishi K, Yoneda R, Tamura M. Difference in the phenotypes of bronchoalveolar lavage lymphocytes in patients with summer-type hypersensitivity pneumonitis, farmer's lung, ventilation pneumonitis, and bird fancier's lung: report of a Nationwide epidemiologic study in Japan. J Allergy Clin Immunol. 1991;87:1002–9. https://doi.org/10.1016/0091-6749(91)90423-l.
4. Banaszak EF, Thiede WH, Fink JN. Hypersensitivity pneumonitis due to contamination of an air conditioner. N Engl J Med. 1970;283:271–6. https://doi.org/10.1097/00043764-197101000-00024.
5. Marinkovich VA, Novey HS. Humidifier lung. Clin Rev Allergy. 1983;1:533–6.
6. Fink JN, Banaszak EF, Theide WH, Barboriak JJ. Interstitial pneumonitis due to hypersensitivity to an organism contaminating a heating system. Ann Intern Med. 1971;74:80–3. https://doi.org/10.7326/0003-4819-74-1-80.
7. Sweet LC, Anderson JA, Callies QC, Coates EO Jr. Hypersensitivity pneumonitis related to a home furnace humidifier. J Allergy Clin lmmunol. 1971;48:171–8. https://doi.org/10.1016/0091-6749(71)90013-3.
8. Fink JN, Banaszak EF, Barboriak JJ, Hensley GT, Kurup VP, Scanlon GT, et al. Interstitial lung disease due to contamination of forced air systems. Ann Intern Med. 1976;84:406–13. https://doi.org/10.7326/0003-4819-84-4-406.
9. Burke GW, Carrington CB, Strauss R, Fink JN, Gaensler EA. Allergic alveolitis caused by home humidifiers. JAMA. 1977;238:2705–8. https://doi.org/10.1001/jama.1977.03280260035013.
10. Robertson AS, Burge PS, Wieland GA, Carmalt MH. Extrinsic allergic alveolitis caused by a cold water humidifier. Thorax. 1987;42:32–7. https://doi.org/10.1136/thx.42.1.32.
11. Suda T, Sato A, Ida M, Gemma H, Hayakawa H, Chida K. Hypersensitivity pneumonitis associated with home ultrasonic humidifiers. Chest. 1995;107:711–7. https://doi.org/10.1378/chest.107.3.711.
12. Nihashi F, Kitahara Y, Murakami Y, Kishimoto Y, Aono Y, Eifuku T, et al. Three cases of humidifier lung associated with respiratory failure. Japan J Sarcoidosis Other Granulomatous Disord. 2018;38:81–4. https://doi.org/10.7878/jjsogd.38.1_2_81.
13. Sakamoto S, Furukawa M, Shimizu H, Muneyuki S, Miyoshi M, et al. Clinical and radiological characteristics of ultrasonic humidifier lung and summer-type hypersensitivity pneumonitis. Respir Med. 2020;174:106196. https://doi.org/10.1164/ajrccm-conference.2021.203.1_meetingabstracts.a1879.
14. Suga M, Yamasaki H, Nakagawa K, Kohrogi H, Ando M, M. Mechanisms accounting for granulomatous response in hypersensitivity pneumonitis. Sarcoidosis Vasc Diffuse Lung Dis. 1997;14:131–8.

15. Flaherty DK, Deck FH, Cooper J, Bishop K, Winzenburger PA, Smith LR, et al. Bacterial endotoxin isolated from a water spray air humidification system as a putative agent of occupation- related lung disease. Infect Immun. 1984;43:206–11. https://doi.org/10.1128/iai.43.1.206-212.1984.
16. Rylander R, Haglind P, Lundholm M, Mattsby I, Stenqvist K. Humidifier fever and endotoxin exposure. Clin Allergy. 1978;8:511–6. https://doi.org/10.1111/j.1365-2222.1978.tb01504.x.
17. Muittari A, Kuusisto P, Sovijarvi A. An epidemic of bath water fever–endotoxin alveolitis? Eur J Respir Dis Suppl. 1982;123:108–16.
18. Rylander R, Haglind P. Airborne endotoxins and humidifier disease. Clin Allergy. 1984;14:109–12. https://doi.org/10.1111/j.1365-2222.1984.tb02197.x.
19. Michel O. Systemic and local airways inflammatory response to endotoxin. Toxicology. 2000;152:25–30. https://doi.org/10.1016/s0300-483x(00)00288-2.
20. Thorn J. The inflammatory response in humans after inhalation of bacterial endotoxin: a review. Inflamm Res. 2001;50:254–61. https://doi.org/10.1007/s000110050751.
21. Holz O, Tan L, Schaumann F, Müller M, Scholl D, Hidi R, et al. Inter- and intrasubject variability of the inflammatory response to segmental endotoxin challenge in healthy volunteers. Pulm Pharmacol Ther. 2015;35:50–9. https://doi.org/10.1016/j.pupt.2015.10.011.
22. Stephens RC, O'Malley CM, Frumento RJ, Mythen MG, Bennett-Guerrero E. Low-dose endotoxin elicits variability in the inflammatory response in healthy volunteers. J Endotoxin Res. 2005;11:207–12. https://doi.org/10.1179/096805105x58661.
23. Schwartz DA. The role of TLR4 in endotoxin responsiveness in humans. J Endotoxin Res. 2001;7:389–93. https://doi.org/10.1179/096805101101532972.
24. Arbour NC, Lorenz E, Schutte BC, Zabner J, Kline JN, Jones M, et al. TLR4 mutations are associated with endotoxin hyporesponsiveness in humans. Nat Genet. 2000;25:187–91. https://doi.org/10.1038/76048.
25. Ohnishi H, Yokoyama A, Hamada H, Manabe S, Ito R, Watanabe A, et al. Humidifier lung: possible contribution of endotoxin-induced lung injury. Intern Med. 2002;41:1179–82. https://doi.org/10.2169/internalmedicine.41.1179.
26. Raghu G, Remy-Jardin M, Ryerson CJ, Myers JL, Kreuter M, Vasakova M, et al. Diagnosis of hypersensitivity pneumonitis in adults. An official ATS/JRS/ALAT clinical practice guideline. Am J Respir Crit Care Med. 2020;202:e36–69. https://doi.org/10.1164/rccm.202005-2032st.
27. Fernández Pérez ER, Travis WD, Lynch DA, Brown KK, Johannson KA, Selman M, et al. Diagnosis and evaluation of hypersensitivity pneumonitis: CHEST guideline and expert panel report. Chest. 2021;160:e97–e156. https://doi.org/10.1016/j.chest.2021.03.066.
28. Shimoda M, Morimoto K, Tanaka Y, Furuuchi K, Osawa T, Yano R, et al. Features of humidifier lung and comparison with summer-type hypersensitivity pneumonitis. Respirology. 2021;26:394–5. https://doi.org/10.1111/resp.14014.
29. Takahashi T, Munakata M, Ohtsuka Y, Satoh-Kamachi A, Sato R, Homma Y, et al. Serum KL-6 concentrations in dairy farmers. Chest. 2000;118:445–50. https://doi.org/10.1378/chest.118.2.445.
30. Leatherman JW, Michael AF, Schwartz BA, Hoidal JR. Lung T cells in hypersensitivity pneumonitis. Ann Intern Med. 1984;100:390–2. https://doi.org/10.7326/0003-4819-100-3-390.
31. Costabel U, Bross KJ, Ruhle KH, Löhr GW, Matthys H. Ia-like antigens on T cells and their subpopulations in pulmonary sarcoidosis and in hypersensitivity pneumonitis: analysis of bronchoalveolar and blood lymphocytes. Am Rev Respir Dis. 1985;131:337–42.
32. Semenzato G, Agostini C, Zambello R, Trentin L, Chilosi M, Pizzolo G, et al. Lung T cells in hypersensitivity pneumonitis: phenotypic and functional analyses. J Immunol. 1986;137:1164–72. https://doi.org/10.4049/jimmunol.137.4.1164.

MIX
Papier aus verantwortungsvollen Quellen
Paper from responsible sources
FSC® C105338

If you have any concerns about our products,
you can contact us on
ProductSafety@springernature.com

In case Publisher is established outside the EU,
the EU authorized representative is:
Springer Nature Customer Service Center GmbH
Europaplatz 3, 69115 Heidelberg, Germany

Printed by Libri Plureos GmbH
in Hamburg, Germany